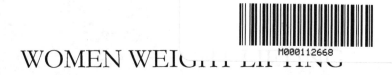

HEAVY
WEIGHTS
TOUGH
WOMEN

*Proven Exercise and Workouts
to Build Lean Muscle and
Strength for the Perfect Female
Body ~ Women's Health*

MIAH ROMERO

Table of Contents

PART I

Chapter 1: Muscle Mass

You have probably heard by now of the many benefits of having more of your body being composed of muscle mass. And yet, I'd venture to guess you still don't know the half of it!

If you're a woman, thirty percent of your body is made up of muscle mass; for men, it's around forty. The bottom line is, we all want more muscle! Muscle gives us that long and lean appearance—with nicely shaped muscles. Muscular people are viewed as healthy people. Obviously, they are also stronger. Too much fat can lead to all kinds of health problems, not to mention all the clothes you have that you can't wear!

There are many, many reasons to desire to build more muscle, but I'll give you the one that is at the top of the list for me: muscle burns fat. That's right! Muscle burns fat not only when you're in the gym or somewhere else, hitting the weights, or doing body resistance training, it does so when you're at rest. That is correct. Muscle eats away at fat while you're lolling on the sofa watching that Sunday afternoon football game.

This is why we love muscle!

Many folks don't do weight training because they think they have to head to the gym. It's a very common myth that it's necessary to use weights in order to add muscle. But it's just that—a myth. You also don't have to purchase a room full of expensive weights, gadgets and other equipment to use to build muscle at home.

I'm going to let you in on a little secret. You can build muscle using just...you. It is true. You can use your own body's resistance against itself to burn fat and build muscle. It's awesome! This way, there are no excuses. You don't have to pay a gym membership, drive yourself there, or even leave the comfort of your own home.

I'm going to give you nine different muscle-building, fat-burning workouts, and we're going to talk—just a little—about a few things you can do in the area of diet. Yes, diet. Not "diet" as in a bad word—like "I feel miserable after eating badly for the last two weeks and I need to go on a diet." Not that sort of talk. We'll simply touch on some of the foods you should be eating and some of the food you shouldn't be if you're genuinely interested in losing some weight.

Before we get into the exercises, let's cover some basics.

1.1. How Muscle is Built

Simply put in laymen's terms, when you work out, you essentially damage your muscles. Muscle tissue is broken down. When this process happens, your body gets busy repairing and replacing these damaged tissues. To get just a little technical during this process, the body has a process on the cellular level in which it repairs or replaces the damaged muscle fibers. It fuses these fibers together to form new myofibrils (muscle protein strands). Repaired myofibrils are larger in thickness and are greater in number, thus causing muscle hypertrophy (growth). This process doesn't happen when you are lifting weights, though. It happens afterward when the body is at rest. That's why rest is absolutely a key component to muscle growth. The hard work is only half the process. But fortunately the rest—pun intended—is easy.

Chapter 2: The Upper Body

"Can we please have a moment of silence for all those stuck in traffic on the way to the gym?" —Anonymous

These aren't always the easiest exercises to do—well, actually, exercising isn't exactly easy anyway, so scratch that. The great thing about upper body work is that this is where you will begin to see results first. So, for that reason, doing upper body work can be incredibly rewarding.

2.1 The Classic Push-Up

Push-ups are super easy, super basic and have been around forever. The reason they've been around forever is that they're also super effective. The key is to perform them correctly. If you don't, they become wasted effort.

2.1.1 The proper way to do push-ups

Get on the ground, belly down. Place your palms on the floor a shoulder width apart or slightly more. Keep your body straight as you push yourself up by extending your arms. Repeat. Make sure that your arms are lifting your body weight, not the muscles on the lower half of your body. Imagine there is a plank of wood on your back starting from your head to your feet. Make sure that your body is as straight as that plank in order to maintain correct body alignment.

2.1.2 How many push-ups?

That depends on the kind of shape you are in when you start. When you begin to do the push-ups, do they feel easy to you? Make sure you are performing the move deliberately—not going too fast that you're using momentum. The first time you try, do as many as you can while still keeping perfect form. Afterward, for your regular sets, do two-thirds that many. So, if you did fifteen but were tired by then and beginning to lose form, use ten as a target for your sets in the beginning.

As you get stronger, make the number higher. You want to continue to be challenged. Some people do as many as one-hundred push-ups per day. Perhaps that's something you can aim for. For the average beginner, three sets of ten are reasonable.

2.2 Chair-Dips

This is another upper-body exercise that, while in actuality, you're using your body-weight, you'll still need a chair or a bench or something similar. When I'm out running, there's a square cement planter that has an edge to it, and it works perfectly.

Dips further work the rhomboid muscles in your back and synchronize with push-ups on working your triceps.

Get a chair/bench or another object capable of supporting your body weight and of a similar height, as explained above. Stand with your back to it. Make sure that the object is sturdy enough to support your entire body weight. Lower yourself and place your palms on the front edge of the bench, fingers pointing forward. Tuck in your elbows to your sides. Maintain this position and walk just your feet slowly in front of you. Your body weight should be resting on your arms now. Deliberately bend your arms and lower yourself. Do this until the floor is parallel to your upper arms. If you're doing it right, you'll feel it in your back and also in your triceps. Simply hold for about a second and return to the starting position.

Do three sets. Determine the number of repetitions per set the exact same way as you did for the push-ups.

2.3 Diamond Push-Ups

Oh, chicken wings—and not the kind you eat. "Chicken wing" is a common term used to refer to the fat on the back of a person's upper arm as it kind of tends to sag, resulting in an unattractive "flapping in the wind" sort of scenario when you wave your arms. Nobody has time for this, people! Not when there are exercises that will blast those wings if you simply stay consistent. Almost everyone wants tight, toned arms. It's a sexy look, and it's youthful! Tight triceps can actually defy a woman's age. So don't skimp on the upper body exercises. I'm giving you three here, and all of them work your triceps, but the Diamond Push-Up works it the most of all so if you're only worried about triceps and nothing else, do this one.

Start in the push-up position, yet instead of having your hands out to the sides, place them in front of you and put them together to create a diamond shape.

Raise yourself until your legs are straight then lower yourself until you are two inches above the ground. You will feel the burn in those triceps. Embrace the burn! The burn means the move is working.

Choose your number of reps in the same manner with all of the upper body exercises.

Chapter 3: The Core

You must not ignore the importance of core work when it comes to resistance training. Your core muscles are the ones that essentially holds everything else together.

There's a very good chance that, no matter what you're doing, you're using your core. Having a weak core takes the power away from all the rest of your muscles. Your core muscles are also responsible for your balance and stability, which is huge. Your core is not one muscle; it's a complicated interconnected series of muscles which effectively include all of them except your arms and your legs. So, I reiterate. Working your core needs to be an incredibly important part of your exercise routine.

Think about your abs. Everybody seems to be concerned with their abdominal muscles. Many people want those six-pack muscles to show. Some just want to button their favorite jeans without lying on the bed.

There's a common misconception (still) that fat can be "spot-burned." This is simply not true. The general consensus is that fat leaves the body the same way it came on—gradually and kind of all over. Don't get me wrong on this; genetics do play a role in how our bodies store fat. Some people can be perfectly proportioned pretty much everywhere on their bodies and yet have large, unattractive bellies. Those people are still more the exception than the rule.

So, the bottom line is that you cannot target fat-burning. If you really want the fat to leave your body, there are three central areas that will require your attention: diet, cardio, and resistance training. Here we are focusing on the third, and a little later I'm going to give a quick overall snapshot of the importance of combining all three.

I'm going to give you three exercises for your core. This first one, known as a Plank, could actually be used as the only core exercise you do. It is that effective and, especially considering the other exercises you'll be doing with, will touch all the muscles in your core.

Now, remember what we said about abs and fat? Here's something many people simply don't realize. Underneath however much fat we happen to be carrying on our abdominal muscles, we all have a "six-pack." Those are muscles in each of our bodies. What people are trying to do when they say they're going for six-pack abs is burn the layers of fat that cover those muscles. As I said, and much to the sadness of myself and many others, you can't target that weight.

Additionally, I'm not going to include any kind of "sit-ups" in upper body work. They've been proven to not be as effective as other exercises that work the core muscles. Also, I personally think that unless your form is always perfect with a sit-up, you may be putting certain back muscles at risk.

3.1 Plank

This one is tough, but like I said, with this one exercise and all the many variations you can do with it, you can get those core muscles strong in no time.

Start with the initial push-up position. Bend your elbows to a right angle. Let your weight rest on your forearms. You might want to get a mat or something soft to use as padding between your arms and the floor. Make sure you have a timer too. The elbows need to be beneath your shoulders directly. Your body should be forming a straight line from head to heels—like a plank. Hold this position for as long as you can without injuring yourself.

Your goal should eventually be to hold it for two minutes. I said eventually for a good reason. Planks are tough. I mean, for a lot of people, a ten-second plank and they're toast. Because so many muscles are used to hold this position, if those muscles aren't strong, it simply can't happen for very long. That's also why planks are such a good indicator of how far you've come. If, when you start it takes all you have to hold a thirty-second plank, I would venture to guess that after a religiously followed routine, within eight weeks you will have worked up to the full two minutes.

Planks are great because there are many variations of them, as well. As you get stronger, try this:

- While in plank position, lift one of your legs as high as you can and hold it there for a count of thirty. Repeat on the other side.
- You can even do a side plank. Lay down on your side with your head propped on your elbow, raise your body in that position and hold it. To increase difficulty with this one, once you are in the up position, try raising your top leg and holding it in that position.

Planks can be thought of as a "Super Move." They literally work all of your muscles. In fact, if one really wanted to, one could do planks only as their resistance training (planks in all their variations, which are many) and achieve the results they're looking for.

3.2   Reverse Crunch

Okay, so I realize I just got done telling you that sit-ups, which are essentially crunches, are not good for the back muscles. In fact, one physician has said that he has seen no other cause of back injury with the highest rate as traditional crunches.

However, the reverse crunch, despite its name, does not carry the same risks and is excellent at targeting your abdominal muscles.

Here's how to do it:

- Lie down on the floor and fully extend your arms and legs to the sides. Put your palms on the floor. Your arms should actually stay in one place as you perform the entire exercise.
- This is the position you will start from: your legs will be pulled up which will make your thighs form a right angle with the floor. You will want your feet together and also parallel to the floor.

- Move your legs towards your torso. At the same time, roll your pelvis backward. Raise your hips above the floor. The goal is to have your knees touching your chest.

- Hold this position for around a second, then lower back to the starting position.

Again, depending on your ability when you start, gauge the number of reps and sets by how they feel to your body and how hard it is for you to do them at first. Just make sure not to overestimate yourself too much. Muscle soreness from overdoing it is no fun!

3.3 Mountain Climber

Get into the top of the push-up position. This is the starting position.

Keeping your back in a straight line, bring your right knee toward your chest. Quickly bring it back to the starting position. Do the same for the left knee. Repeat but speed up the movement, alternating legs quickly as if you were running in place with your hands on the ground.

As far as how many sets, this move isn't exactly structured that way so use seconds to guide you. Try the move until you are really struggling to continue (you'll likely be out of breath) then use two-thirds of those seconds, call it a set, and do three.

Chapter 4: The Lower Body

Working out your lower body is not to be taken lightly or skimped on when doing resistance training. One particular reason for this is because your lower body contains the largest muscle in your entire body: the gluteus maximus.

Not only do most of us like to work out this muscle because it makes us "look" better, it's also a powerhouse. This muscle, along with other gluteal muscles, is one of the great stabilizers of the human body. Keeping these muscles strong can minimize aches and pains in your lower back and hips. The muscles also give you the power you need to do simple things like walk, run, and climb.

So, whenever lower body resistance training is discussed, there are two moves that are practically givens. No, it's not because they're both somewhat torturous—it's because they are effective!

When you're doing your workout, never forget the old adage, "Pain is temporary…(fill in the blank)." Usually, people say, "pain is temporary, quitting lasts forever."

That doesn't exactly apply here, but the point is that if you aren't going to be able to tolerate a little bit of pain, you aren't going to get the same results. Workouts can hurt. Muscles burn. Sometimes by the end of a good workout, you feel like you're about to croak. As far as I'm concerned, those are the very best kind! It means you've really kicked some gluteal maximuses and made some progress for the day. You have to maintain a good attitude if you're going to embark on this journey. Results don't happen overnight, but relatively you will start to see them very quickly (although, in general people who are close to you will notice before you do.) However, nothing is more satisfying than when you do look in the mirror and see results that can't be denied, or when you put on a pair of jeans that has been an eternity since they were last wore and they button easily. It's a powerful feeling.

So, here they come, the not-always-fun but ever-so-productive lower body movements.

4.1 The Lunge

If you've ever done them, you're probably feeling the burn simply at the thought! When executed correctly, these babies do burn, but they are incredibly effective.

Lunges produce fast results. You will notice that your legs and derriere are more toned and attractive looking. You will feel that you're stronger and you'll notice the difference when you do cardio—assuming you do, of course.

Lunges do not require weights, although weights can be added later on to increase the difficulty as you get into better shape.

Form in lunges is very important. The same is true with all of these exercises. If you're going to put in the effort, you may as well make sure you're doing it right in order to maximize your results.

Following is how to execute a perfect lunge:

- Stand upright and keep your body straight. Pull your shoulders back and relax your chin. Keep your chin pointed forward, don't look down. Make sure the muscles in your core are tight and engaged.
- If it helps you with balance, you can use something you have on hand, like, say, a broom. Hold it crossways in front of you and let it lightly rest on your shoulders.

- Pick a leg. Step forward using that leg. Lower your hips until both your knees are forming a right angle. Make sure that your lowered knee isn't touching the floor and that your forward knee is directly above your angle and not too far forward. Make sure that your weight is in your heels as you push yourself back up to the starting position.

- When you do push back up to the starting position, really place extra emphasis on engaging your gluteus maximus. Deliberately use the strength in that muscle to push yourself upright.

Now. Repeat. How many times? I recommend starting with three sets of ten perfectly executed lunges. If you don't feel "the burn" add a couple, or go ahead and use a barbell if you have one and put some weight on it. You can even do lunges in reverse, to vary things up.

4.2 Squat

Ah, the squat. If you haven't done them, you've probably heard of them if you have any friends at all who work out. Like lunges, they are simple, easy to execute, and incredibly effective at increasing muscle mask and making you stronger.

Also, like lunges, there are quite a few variations to squats that you can use as you get more fit. For now, of course, we'll focus on the simple squat. Again, form is super important.

Stand with your feet at least shoulder-width apart. If you feel more comfortable, it's okay to place your feet a bit wider apart. As you stand, you should focus on having your weight on your heels. Extend your arms straight out. The first thing you'll do is thrust your hips back slightly as though you are about to take a seat. Then, lower yourself down like that as if you are actually about to sit down. You'll want to go as low as you can. The goal is to make your knees bent so that your legs are parallel to the floor, again almost if you were sitting in a chair. Control your knees so they don't move forward over your feet.

The next step is simply to stand up, and when you are coming upright, squeeze your glutes at the top of the movement. So, essentially, squats are like sitting in an invisible chair, then standing up using your glutes to propel you. Very easy but super effective!

4.3   The Bridge

The bridge is another great one for strengthening your glutes and legs. Remember, before you even see the results of these exercises, you'll be stronger for doing them. And, if you eat right and take in enough protein (building blocks for muscle) you will increase the size of your muscle and consequently burn fat. So when you're doing these not-so-fun-at-the-time moves, keep that in mind!

Here's how to do a bridge: Lie on the floor, flat as a pancake. Place your hands on your sides and bend your knees. Your feet should be about shoulder-width apart. Lift your hips off the floor, using your heels to push. Keep your back straight while doing this! Hold the position for a second and squeeze those glutes.

Slowly lower back to the position you started from.

For the number of reps, use the method we discussed previously. The first time you try the exercise, go until you really feel the burn—until it's very tough to continue or until you would not be able to. However many reps that is (say it's fifteen) subtract one-third of that number and start from there.

For variety, this exercise can be performed with one leg at a time.

Chapter 5: Putting it all Together

People have different preferences in how they like to work out. To see good results from strength training, you need to work each muscle group no less than two times per week. Three times is fine and you may see faster results that way. Depending on what you want to accomplish, generally, three times is enough.

The idea is to give each muscle group a rest day in between your workouts. So people go about the entire construct differently. Some like to work their entire body in one session, then rest for a day or two and do it again, up to three times a week.

Others prefer to break the muscle group workouts up. Legs one day, arms the next, core the next, like that.

In my opinion and in consideration of the research I've done, any of the above-mentioned ways to go about it will be just as effective as another. Of course, the most important component is that it gets done.

I'd like to take a moment at the time to talk about cardiovascular workouts. I know, I know, boo, hiss. A lot of people really aren't that big on cardio. However, there's a lot to be said for a good cardio sweat session. For one thing, cardiovascular exercise improves the health of our heart and lungs. That alone should be reason enough to work some in. Also, this type of exercise, depending on the type you choose, can burn an awful lot of calories. Remember, any calories burned will contribute to that sleek, muscular look. For the muscles to come out, the fat has to come off.

Cardiovascular exercise has also been proven to affect our moods in a positive way (the same can be said for weight training.)

The best, most well-rounded exercise plans include a mixture of both. Supposing you hate cardio, you will do yourself no harm by keeping it to a minimum. The general recommendation right now is to get thirty minutes of cardio on "most" days of the week.

Given that, as an example, you could do your weights on Monday, cardio Tuesday, weights Wednesday, Cardio Thursday, weights Friday and guess what? Take the weekend off!

This is just one example of how this can all be done. You can be as creative as you want to be or as you need to be to get around a work schedule.

You could do, for instance, cardio in the morning and resistance training at night. You could work in all or part of your resistance training during your lunch hour at work.

There are no limits to the options available, so that simply means *no excuses*.

No equipment or anything fancy is required for the cardio portion either. Walking is cardio. Just walk fast enough to get your heart rate up, break a sweat and breathe a little heavy. Increase intensity as your fitness level improves.

Here's a sample plan, if you need one. I'm going to use ten reps as a standard while performing the strength training for the sake of simplicity.

Monday Morning Before Work:

Three sets of ten of each of the following:

- Push-ups
- Chair-Dips
- Diamond Push-ups

Honestly, this should take you no more than ten minutes.

Monday Lunch:

- Walk for thirty minutes

Monday Evening:

Perform three sets of the following:

- Squats
- Lunges
- Bridges
- Planks
- Mountain Climber
- Reverse Crunch

Starting out, repeat this same routine on Wednesdays and Fridays. Try this for a few weeks (or another plan of your own design) and see how it works with your schedule.

On the days that you don't walk for thirty-minutes on your lunch, per your official "schedule," do it anyway. If not that, jump on the trampoline with your little ones at night for half an hour. Ride your bike. Swim. Ski if you live near snow and/or if it's wintertime. Snow Show. Or...head to the gym. Do the elliptical or the stair-climber for half of an hour. It's really not hard to get in the minimum amount of cardio and depending on your goals, and who says you have to stop with the minimum?

If you stick to this program, you're going to see some results and you'll see them pretty quickly.

Here's another tip: throw away your scale. Okay, well you don't have to throw it away. I just don't recommend weighing yourself all the time. It could discourage you in fact, for the simple reason that muscle actually does weigh more than fat. You might gain in the beginning, and no one wants to start a workout program only to see the numbers on the scale go up. No way! Instead of worrying about the scale, judge your progress by—most importantly—how you feel, and as for changes in your body, you can always take some initial measurements and then re-measure once a week. What has always worked best for me is simply to gauge how my clothes fit. That's the biggest tell of all. I have a pair of jean shorts I'm wearing right now. A couple of months ago I couldn't get them to even think about zipping! That's the only kind of progress I need. To me, numbers on the scale don't mean a whole lot.

Chapter 6: On Your Diet

It wouldn't be right to talk about gaining muscle and losing fat without talking a bit about diet.

I'm not going to go overboard but there are a few things I'd like to touch on.

First off, as I previously spoke about at the end of chapter four—the scale—I forgot to mention another reason I don't care to use them. Most of them have a tendency to fluctuate as much as five pounds in less than twenty-four hours. In other words, if I'm going by the scale, I often will have "gained" five pounds from when I got up to when it's time for bed.

Not cool.

Not possible, either. Our bodies are made up of an estimated sixty-five percent water. It is normal for the amount of water in our bodies to fluctuate all the time. Losing water weight does not equate to losing fat. However, while we are trying to lose weight, and while we're working out, it is especially important to keep our bodies hydrated.

There are as many theories on the web as you could click on about how much water to drink, but for questions like these, I like to refer to the Mayo Clinic website, because I know that the information they put out there has been thoroughly researched. What follows is their advice on water intake:

Every single day, you lose water by breathing, sweating, urinating, and pooping. To function properly, your body's water must be replenished through the consumption of food and beverages.

The average healthy man who lives in a temperate climate needs 15.5 cups or 3.7 liters of fluids every day, and the average healthy woman living in the same place needs 11.5 cups or 2.7 liters every day.

This is about what I do for myself in a normal day and it seems to work. Regardless, don't skimp on the water.

There's another important factor when it comes to building muscle and that is protein. If you are serious about adding some muscle mass, you're going to need to eat your protein. That doesn't mean it has to be meat; there are plenty of non-meat options for protein intake. Of course, if you are a vegetarian you already know that.

Another little tip: your body needs fat to lose fat. Sounds strange, doesn't it? But if your body is starved of nutrients, it will begin to hold on to everything it has instinctually, and as a result, you won't see any weight loss.

There are a million types of "diets" out there, and this is not a book about diets so I'm not going to delve into them. If I were going to say anything at all about your diet (and don't get me wrong, your diet IS important,) I would say two words: eat clean.

What does that mean? Since clean is the opposite of dirty, in this case, think dirty equals "processed."

Do your body a giant favor and stay away from processed foods! Eat foods that are as "close" to the earth as you can.

- Lean proteins (including fish and non-meat proteins)
- Tons—and I do really mean tons—of vegetables
- Lean fat (avocado, almonds, coconut oil)
- Dairy (full-fat; eat sparingly)
- Fruits (sparingly)

It's that simple. No "TV Dinners." No boxes of macaroni and cheese, please. Nothing that has a "bunch" of ingredients, many of which you aren't even familiar with. Those are bad. Leave them in the store.

If you have a sweet tooth, indulge it, but rarely, and even a sweet tooth can be indulged in a healthy manner. There's nothing wrong with eating some strawberries topped with full fat whipped cream. Yummy!

Well, there you have it. You really are set. Everything is explained and condensed for you.

Start your weight training and your cardio, eat clean, drink your water and reap the rewards.

Go get 'em!

PART II

Chapter 1: Meal Planning 101

Sticking to a diet is something that is not the easiest in the world. When it comes down to it, we struggle to change up our diets on a whim. It might be that for the first few days, you are able to stick to it and make sure that you are only eating those foods that are better for you, but over time, you will get to a point where you feel the pressure to cave in. You might realize that sticking to your diet is difficult and think that stopping for a burger on your way home won't be too bad. You might think that figuring out lunch or dinner is too much of a hassle, or you realize that the foods that you have bought forgot a key ingredient that you needed for dinner.

The good news is, you have an easy fix. When you are able to figure out what you are making for yourself for your meals well in advance, you stop having to worry so much about the foods that you eat, what you do with them, and what you are going to reach for when it's time to eat. You will be able to change up what you are doing so that you can be certain that the meals that you are enjoying are good for you, and you won't have to worry so much about the stress that goes into it. Let's take a look at what you need to do to get started with meal planning so that you can begin to do so without having to think too much about it.

Make a Menu

First, before you do anything, make sure that you make a menu! This should be something that you do on your own, or you should sit down with your family to ask them what they prefer. If you can do this, you will be able to ensure that you've got a clear-cut plan. When you have a menu a week in advance, you save yourself time and money because you know that all of your meals will use ingredients that are similar, and you won't have to spend forever thinking about what you should make at any point in time.

Plan around Ads

When you do your menu, make it a point to glance through the weekly ads as well. Typically, you will find that there are plenty of deals that you can make use of that will save you money.

Go Meatless Once Per Week

A great thing to do that is highly recommended on the Mediterranean Diet is to have a day each week where you go meatless for dinner. By doing so, you will realize that you can actually cut costs and enjoy the foods more at the same time. It is a great way to get that additional fruit and veggie content into your day, and there are plenty of healthy options that are out there for you. You just have to commit to doing so. In the meal plans that you'll see below, you will notice that there will be a meatless day on Day 2 every week.

Use Ingredients That You Already Have On Hand

Make it a point to use ingredients that you already have on hand whenever possible. Alternatively, make sure that all of the meals that you eat during the week use very similar ingredients. When you do this, you know that you're avoiding causing any waste or losing ingredients along the way, meaning that you can save money. The good news is, on the Mediterranean diet, there are plenty of delicious meals that enjoy very similar ingredients that you can eat.

Avoid Recipes that Call for a Special Ingredient

If you're trying to avoid waste, it is a good idea for you to avoid any ingredients in meals that are not going to carry over to other meals during your weekly plan. By avoiding doing so, you can usually save yourself that money for that one ingredient that would be wasted. Alternatively, if you find that you really want that dish, try seeing if you can freeze some of it for later. When you do that, you can usually ensure that your special ingredient at least didn't go to waste.

Use Seasonal Foods

Fruits and veggies are usually cheaper when you buy them in season, and even better, when you do so, you will be enjoying a basic factor of the Mediterranean diet just by virtue of enjoying the foods when they are fresh. Fresher foods are usually tastier, and they also tend to carry more vitamins and minerals because they have not had the chance to degrade over time.

Make Use of Leftovers and Extra Portions

One of the greatest things that you can do when it comes to meal planning is to make use of your leftovers and make-ahead meals. When you do this regularly, making larger portions than you need, you can then use the extras as lunches and dinners all week long, meaning that you won't have to be constantly worrying about the food that you eat for lunch. We will use some of these in the meal plans that you will see as well.

Eat What You Enjoy

Finally, the last thing to remember with your meal plan is that you ought to be enjoying the foods that are on it at all times. When you ensure that the foods that you have on your plate are those that you actually enjoy, sticking to your meal plan doesn't become such a chore, and that means that you will be able to do better as well with your own diet. Your meal plan should be loaded up with foods that you are actually excited about enjoying. Meal planning and dieting should not be a drag—you should love every moment of it!

Chapter 2: 1 Month Meal Plan

This meal plan is designed to be used for one month to help you simplify making sure that you have delicious meals to eat without having to think. These meals are fantastic options if you don't know where to start but want to enjoy your Mediterranean diet without much hassle. For each of the five weeks included, you will get one breakfast recipe, one lunch recipe, one dinner recipe, and one snack recipe to make meal planning a breeze. So, give these recipes a try! Many of them are so delicious, you'll want to enjoy them over and over again!

Week 1: Success is no accident—you have to reach for it

Mediterranean Breakfast Sandwich

Serves: 4

Time: 20 minutes

Ingredients:

- Baby spinach (2 c.)

- Eggs (4)

- Fresh rosemary (1 Tbsp.)

- Low-fat feta cheese (4 Tbsp.)

- Multigrain sandwich thins (4)

- Olive oil (4 tsp.)

- Salt and pepper according to preference

- Tomato (1, cut into 8 slices)

Instructions:

1. Preheat your oven. This recipe works best at 375° F. Cut the sandwich things in half and brush the insides with half of your olive oil. Place the things on a baking sheet and toast for about five minutes or until the edges are lightly browned and crispy.

2. In a large skillet, heat the rest of your olive oil and the rosemary. Use medium-high heat. Crack your eggs into the skillet one at a time. Cook until the whites have set while keeping the yolks runny. Break the yolks and flip the eggs until done.

3. Serve by placing spinach in between two sandwich thins, along with two tomato slices, an egg, and a tablespoon of feta cheese.

Greek Chicken Bowls

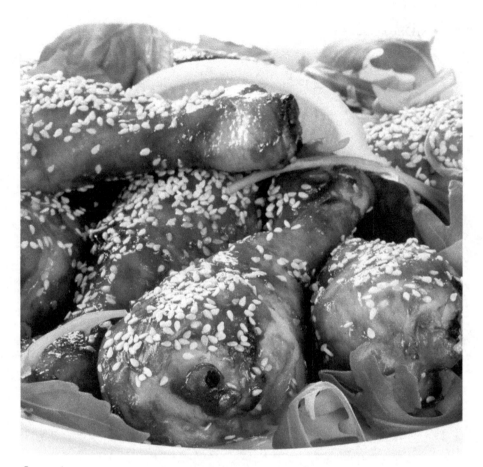

Serves: 4

Time: 20 minutes

Ingredients:

- Arugula (4 c.)
- Chicken breast tenders (1 lb.)

- Cucumber (1, diced)
- Curry powder (1 Tbsp.)
- Dried basil (1 tsp.)
- Garlic powder (1 tsp.)
- Kalamata olives (2 Tbsp.)
- Olive oil (1 Tbsp.)
- Pistachios (0.25 c., chopped)
- Red onion (half, sliced)
- Sunflower seeds (0.25 c.)
- Tzatziki sauce (1 c.)

Instructions:

1. In a bowl, mix in the chicken tenders, curry powder, dried basil, and garlic powder. Make sure to coat the chicken evenly.
2. Heat one tablespoon of olive oil over medium-high. Add the chicken and cook for about four minutes on each side. Remove from the pan and set aside to cool.
3. Place one cup of arugula into four bowls. Toss in the diced cucumber, onion, and kalamata olives.
4. Chop the chicken and distribute evenly between the four bowls.
5. Top with tzatziki sauce, pistachio seeds, and sunflower seeds.

Ratatouille

Serves: 8

Time: 1 hour 30 minutes

Ingredients:

- Crushed tomatoes (1 28 oz. can)
- Eggplants (2)
- Fresh basil (4 Tbsp., chopped)
- Fresh parsley (2 Tbsp., chopped)
- Fresh thyme (2 tsp.)
- Garlic cloves (4, minced and 1 tsp, minced)
- Olive oil (6 Tbsp.)
- Onion (1, diced)
- Red bell pepper (1, diced)
- Roma tomatoes (6)
- Salt and pepper to personal preference
- Yellow bell pepper (1, diced)
- Yellow squashes (2)
- Zucchinis (2)

Instructions:

1. Get your oven ready. This recipe works best at 375° F.
2. Slice the tomatoes, eggplant, squash, and zucchini into thin rounds and set them to the side.

3. Heat up two tablespoons of olive oil in an oven safe pan using medium-high heat. Sauté your onions, four cloves of garlic, and bell peppers for about ten minutes or when soft. Add in your pepper and salt along with the full can of crushed tomatoes. Add in two tablespoons of basil. Stir thoroughly.

4. Take the vegetable slices from earlier and arrange them on top of the sauce in a pattern of your choosing. For example, a slice of eggplant, followed by a slice of tomato, squash, and zucchini, then repeating. Start from the outside and work inward to the center of your pan. Sprinkle salt and pepper overtop the veggies.

5. In a bowl, toss in the remaining basil and garlic, thyme, parsley, salt, pepper, and the rest of the olive oil. Mix it all together, and spoon over the veggies.

6. Cover your pan and bake for 40 minutes. Uncover and then continue baking for another 20 minutes.

Snack Platter

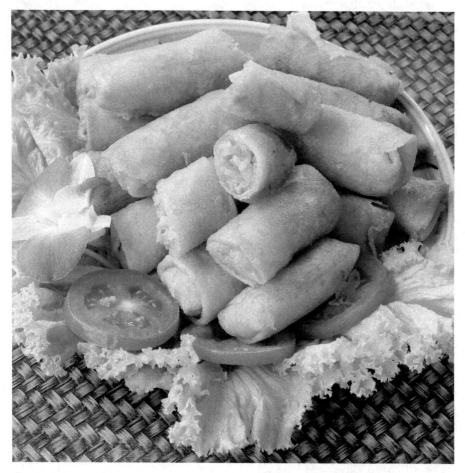

Serves: 6

Time:

Ingredients:

Rosemary Almonds

- Butter (1 Tbsp.)

- Dried rosemary (2 tsp.)
- Salt (pinch)
- Whole almonds (2 c.)

Hummus

- Chickpeas (1 15 oz. can, drained and rinsed)
- Garlic clove (1, peeled)
- Lemon (half, juiced)
- Olive oil (2 Tbsp.)
- Salt and pepper according to personal preference
- Tahini (2 Tbsp.)
- Water (2 Tbsp.)

Other sides

- Bell pepper (1, sliced)
- Cucumber (1, sliced)
- Feta cheese (4 oz, cubed)
- Kalamata olives (handful, drained)
- Pepperoncini peppers (6, drained)
- Pitas (6, sliced into wedges)
- Small fresh mozzarella balls (18)
- Soppressata (6 oz.)
- Sweet cherry peppers (18)

Instructions:

1. To get started, make your rosemary almonds. Take a large skillet and place it on a burner set to medium heat. Start melting the butter in, then toss in the almonds, rosemary and a bit of salt. Toss the nuts on occasion to ensure even coating.

2. Cook the almonds for roughly ten minutes, getting them nicely toasted. Set the almonds off to the side to let them cool.

3. Now you'll set out to make the hummus. Take a blender or food processor and toss in the hummus ingredients. Blend until you get a nice, smooth paste. If you find that your paste is too thick, try blending in a bit of water until you get the desired consistency. Once you have the right consistency, taste for seasoning and adjust as necessary.

4. Pour and scrape the hummus into a bowl and drizzle in a bit of olive oil. Set it off to the side to get the rest of the platter going.

5. Grab the sweet cherry peppers and stuff them with the little balls of mozzarella. Arrange a platter in any pattern you like. If serving for a party or family, try keeping each snack in its own little segment to keep things looking neat.

Week 2: Self-belief and effort will take you to what you want to achieve

Breakfast Quesadilla

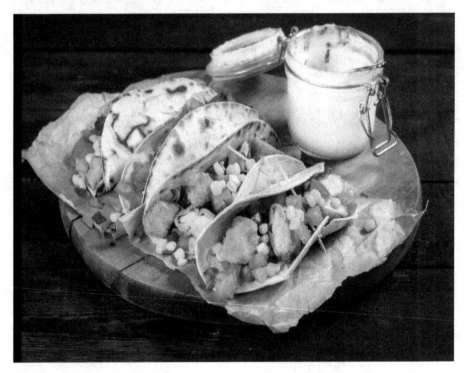

Serves: 1

Time: 10 minutes

Ingredients:

- Basil (handful)
- Eggs (2)
- Flour tortilla (1)

- Green pesto (1 tsp.)
- Mozzarella (0.25 c.)
- Salt and pepper according to personal preference
- Tomato (half, sliced)

Instructions:

1. Scramble your eggs until just a little runny. Remember, you will be cooking them further inside the quesadilla. Season with salt and pepper.
2. Take the eggs and spread over half of the tortilla.
3. Add basil, pesto, mozzarella cheese, and the slices of tomato.
4. Fold your tortilla and toast on an oiled pan. Toast until both sides are golden brown.

Greek Orzo Salad

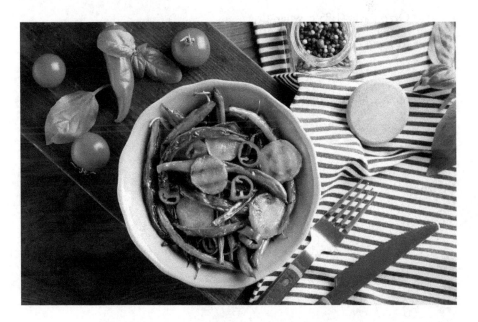

Serves: 6

Time: 25 minutes

Ingredients:

- Canned chickpeas (1 c., drained and rinsed)
- Dijon mustard (0.5 tsp)
- Dill (0.33 c., chopped)
- Dried oregano (1 tsp)
- English cucumber (half, diced)
- Feta cheese crumbles (0.5 c.)
- Kalamata olives (0.33 c., halved)
- Lemon (half, juice and zest)
- Mint (0.33 c., chopped)
- Olive oil (3 Tbsp.)
- Orzo pasta (1.25 c. when dry)
- Roasted red pepper (half, diced)
- Salt and pepper to taste
- Shallot (0.25 c., minced)
- White wine vinegar (2 Tbsp.)

Instructions:

1. Prepare the orzo according to the packaging details. Once the orzo is al dente, drain it and rinse until it drops to room temperature.
2. In a bowl, toss all the ingredients together until thoroughly incorporated.

One Pot Mediterranean Chicken

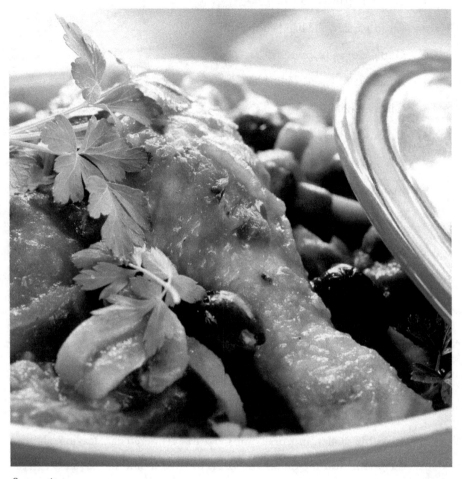

Serves: 4

Time: 1 hour

Ingredients:

- Chicken broth (3 c.)
- Chicken thighs (3, bone in, skin on)

- Chickpeas (1 15 oz can, drained and rinsed)

- Dried oregano (0.5 tsp.)

- Fresh parsley (2 Tbsp., chopped)

- Garlic cloves (2, minced)

- Kalamata olives (0.75 c., halved)

- Olive oil (2 tsp.)

- Onion (1, finely diced)

- Orzo pasta (8 ounces uncooked)

- Roasted peppers (0.5 c., chopped)

- Salt and pepper according to personal preference

Instructions:

1. Prepare your oven at 375°. Heat your olive oil in a large skillet over medium-high heat.
2. Season the chicken with salt and pepper on both sides. Toss the chicken into the skillet and cook for five minutes on each side, or until golden in color. Remove the chicken.
3. Take the skillet and drain most of the rendered fat, leaving about a teaspoon. Add the onion and cook for five minutes. Toss in the garlic and cook for an additional minute.
4. Now you will want to add the orzo, roasted peppers, oregano, chickpeas, and olives into the pan. Add in salt and pepper.
5. Place the thighs on top of the orzo and pour in the chicken broth.
6. Bring to a boil, then cover and place in the oven. Bake for 35 minutes or until chicken has cooked through. Top with parsley and serve.

Mediterranean Nachos

Serves: 6

Time: 10 minutes

Ingredients:

- Canned artichoke hearts (1 c., rinsed, drained, and dried)
- Canned garbanzo beans (0.75 c., rinsed, drained, and dried)
- Feta cheese (0.5 c., crumbled)
- Fresh cilantro (2 Tbsp., chopped)
- Pine nuts (2.5 Tbsp.)
- Roasted red peppers (0.5 c., dried)
- Sabra Hummus (half of their 10 oz. container)
- Tomatoes (0.5 c., chopped)
- Tortilla chips (roughly half a bag)

Instructions:

1. Get your oven ready by setting it to 375°F. In a baking pan, layer the tortilla chips, and spread hummus over them evenly. Top with garbanzo beans, red peppers, artichoke hearts, feta cheese, and pine nuts.
2. Bake for about five minutes or until warmed through. Remove the baking pan and top the nachos with fresh cilantro and tomatoes. Serve and enjoy.

Week 3: The harder you work, the greater the success

Breakfast Tostadas

Serves: 4

Time: 15 minutes

Ingredients:

- Beaten eggs (8)
- Cucumber (0.5 c., seeded and chopped)
- Feta (0.25 c., crumbled)
- Garlic powder (0.5 tsp)
- Green onions (0.5 c., chopped)
- Oregano (0.5 tsp)
- Red Pepper (0.5 c., diced)
- Roasted red pepper hummus (0.5 c.)
- Skim milk (0.5 c.)
- Tomatoes (0.5 c., diced)
- Tostadas (4)

Instructions:

1. In a large skillet, cook the red pepper for two minutes on medium heat until softened. Toss in the eggs, garlic powder, milk, oregano, and green onions. Stir constantly until the egg whites have set.
2. Top the tostadas with hummus, egg mixture, cucumber, feta, and tomatoes.

Roasted Vegetable Bowl

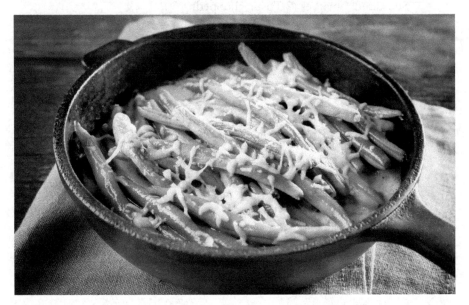

Serves: 2

Time: 45 minutes

Ingredients:

- Crushed red pepper flakes (a pinch)
- Fresh parsley (1 Tbsp., chopped)
- Kalamata olives (0.25 c.)
- Kale (1 c., ribboned)
- Lemon juice (1 Tbsp.)
- Marinated artichoke hearts (0.25 c., drained and chopped)
- Nutritional yeast (1 Tbsp.)
- Olive oil (1 Tbsp., then enough to drizzle)
- Salt and pepper to taste

- Spaghetti squash (half, seeds removed)
- Sun-dried tomatoes (2 Tbsp., chopped)
- Walnuts (0.25 c., chopped)

Instructions:

1. Get your oven ready by setting it to 400° F. Take a baking sheet and blanket it with parchment paper.
2. Take the squash half and place it on the parchment paper. Drizzle olive oil over the side that is cut, and season with salt and pepper. Turn it over so it is facing cut side down and bake for 40 minutes. It is ready when it is soft.
3. Remove the squash shell, and season with a bit more salt and pepper.
4. Stack the kale, artichoke hearts, walnuts, sun-dried tomatoes, and kalamata olives on the squash.
5. Squeeze the lemon juice over and drizzle olive oil. Finish with chopped parsley and a bit of crushed red pepper flakes.

Mediterranean Chicken

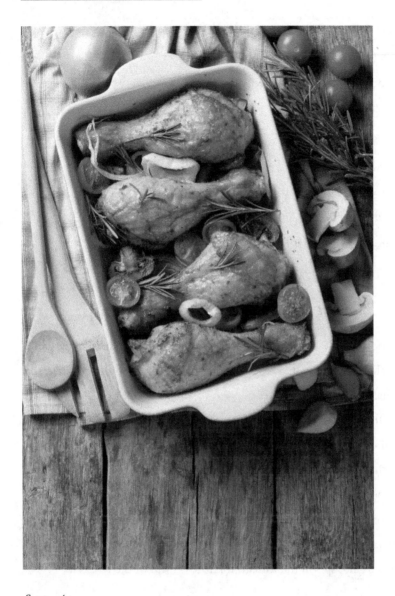

Serves: 4

Time: 40 minutes

Ingredients:

- Chicken breasts (1 lb., boneless, skinless)
- Chives (2 Tbsp., chopped)
- Feta cheese (0.25 c., crumbled)
- Garlic (1 tsp., minced)
- Italian seasoning (1 tsp.)
- Lemon juice (2 Tbsp.)
- Olive oil (2 Tbsp., and 1 Tbsp.)
- Salt and pepper according to personal preference
- Tomatoes (1 c., diced)

Instructions:

1. Pour in two tablespoons of olive oil, the lemon juice, salt, pepper, garlic, and Italian seasoning in a resealable plastic bag. Add in the chicken, seal and shake to coat the chicken.
2. Allow the chicken to marinate for at least 30 minutes in the refrigerator.
3. Heat the rest of the olive oil in a pan over medium heat.
4. Place the chicken on the pan and cook for five minutes on each side, or until cooked through.
5. In a bowl, mix the tomatoes, chives, and feta cheese. Season with salt and pepper.
6. When serving, spoon the tomato mixture on top of the chicken.

Baked Phyllo Chips

Serves: 2

Time: 10 minutes

Ingredients:

- Grated cheese (your choice)
- Olive oil (enough to brush with)
- Phyllo sheets (4)
- Salt and pepper according to personal preference

Instructions:

1. Get your oven ready by setting it to 350° F. Brush olive oil over a phyllo sheet generously. Sprinkle grated cheese and your seasoning on top.
2. Grab a second sheet of your phyllo and place it on top of the first one. Again, brush with olive oil and sprinkle cheese and seasoning on top.
3. Repeat this process with the remaining sheets of phyllo. Top the stack with cheese and seasoning.
4. Once complete, cut the stack of phyllo into bite-sized rectangles. A pizza cutter may be helpful here.
5. Grab a baking sheet and blanket it with some parchment paper. Take your phyllo rectangles and place them on the parchment paper.
6. Bake in the oven for about seven minutes or until they reach a golden color.
7. Remove them from the oven and allow them to cool before serving.

Week 4: You don't need perfection—you need effort

Mini Omelets

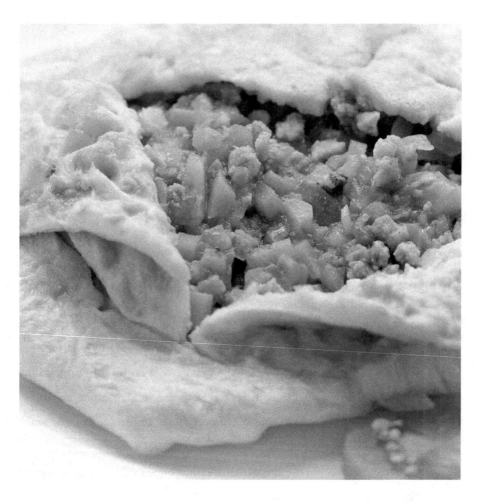

Serves: 8

Time: 40 minutes

Ingredients:

- Cheddar cheese (0.25 c., shredded)
- Eggs (8)
- Half and half (0.5 c.)
- Olive oil (2 tsps.)
- Salt and pepper according to personal preference
- Spinach (1 c., chopped)

Instructions:

1. Get your oven ready by setting it to 350° F. Prepare a muffin pan or ramekins by greasing them with olive oil.
2. In a bowl, beat the eggs and dairy until you have a fluffy consistency.
3. Stir in the cheese and your seasonings. Pour in the spinach and continue beating the eggs.
4. Pour the egg mixture into your ramekins or muffin pan.
5. Bake the omelets until they have set, which should be roughly 25 minutes. Remove them from the oven and allow them to cool before serving.

Basil Shrimp Salad

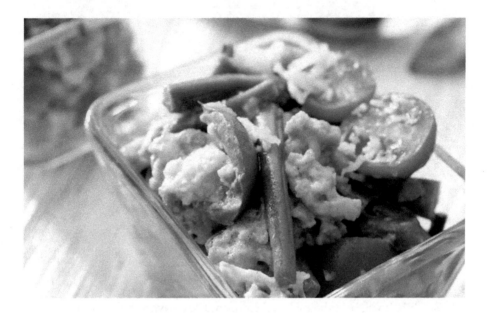

Serves: 2

Time: 40 minutes

Ingredients:

- Dried basil (1 tsp.)
- Lemon juice (1 Tbsp.)
- Olive oil (1 tsp.)
- Romaine lettuce (2 c.)
- Shrimp (12 medium or 8 large)
- White wine vinegar (0.25 c.)

Instructions:

1. Whisk together the white wine vinegar, olive oil, lemon juice, and basil. Stick your shrimp in the marinade for half an hour.
2. Take the marinade and shrimp and cook in a skillet over medium heat until cooked through.
3. Allow the shrimp to cool along with the juice and pour into a bowl. Toss in the romaine lettuce and mix well to get the flavor thoroughly infused in the salad. Serve.

Mediterranean Flounder

Serves: 4

Time: 40 minutes

Ingredients:

- Capers (0.25 c.)
- Diced tomatoes (1 can)
- Flounder fillets (1 lb.)
- Fresh basil (12 leaves, chopped)
- Fresh parmesan cheese (3 Tbsp., grated)
- Garlic cloves (2, chopped)
- Italian seasoning (a pinch)
- Kalamata olives (0.5 c., pitted and chopped)
- Lemon juice (1 tsp.)

- Red onion (half, chopped)
- White wine (0.25 c.)

Instructions:

1. Set your oven to 425° F. Take a skillet and pour in enough olive oil to sauté the onion until soft. Cook on medium-high heat.
2. Toss in the garlic, Italian seasoning, and tomatoes. Cook for an additional five minutes.
3. Pour in the wine, capers, olives, lemon juice, and only half of the basil you chopped.
4. Reduce the heat to low and stir in the parmesan cheese. Simmer for ten minutes or until the sauce has thickened.
5. Place the flounder fillets in a baking pan and pour the sauce over top. Sprinkle the remaining basil on top and bake for 12 minutes.

Nutty Energy Bites

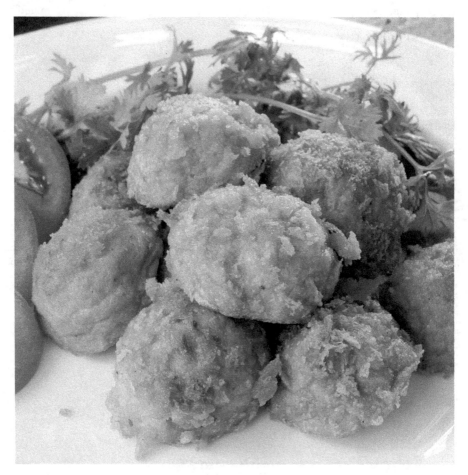

Serves: 10

Time: 10 minutes

Ingredients:

- Dried dates (1 c., pitted)
- Almonds (0.5 c.)

- Pine nuts (0.25 c.)
- Flaxseeds (1 Tbsp., milled) Porridge oats (2 Tbsp.)
- Pistachios (0.25 c., coarsely ground)

Instructions:

1. Take the dates, pine nuts, milled flaxseeds, almonds, and porridge oats and pour them into a food processor or blender. Mix until thoroughly incorporated.
2. Using a tablespoon, scoop the mixture and roll it between your hands until you have a small, bite-sized ball. Do this until you have used the entirety of the dough. This recipe should be enough for about ten.
3. On a plate, sprinkle your ground pistachios. Take the energy balls and roll them on the pistachio grounds, making sure to coat them evenly. Serve or store in the refrigerator.

Week 5: Transformation Happens One Day at a Time

Mediterranean Breakfast Bowl

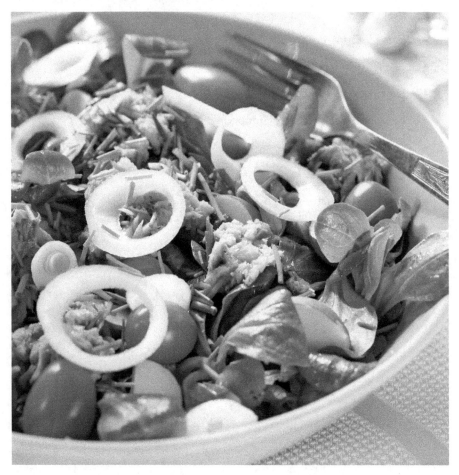

Serves: 1

Time: 25 minutes

Ingredients:

- Artichoke hearts (0.25 c., chopped)
- Baby arugula (2 c.)
- Capers (1 Tbsp.)
- Egg (1)
- Feta (2 Tbsp., crumbled)
- Garlic (0.25 tsp)
- Kalamata olives (5, chopped)
- Lemon thyme (1 Tbsp., chopped)
- Olive oil (0.5 Tbsp.)
- Pepper (0.25 tsp)
- Sun-dried tomatoes (2 Tbsp., chopped)
- Sweet potato (1 c., cubed)

Instructions:

1. Take your olive oil and, when hot, pan fry your sweet potatoes for 5-10 minutes until they have softened. Then, sprinkle on the seasonings.
2. Place arugula into a bowl, then top with potatoes, then everything but the egg.
3. Prepare the egg to your liking and serve.

Chicken Shawarma Pita Pockets

Serves: 6

Time: 40 minutes

Ingredients:

- Cayenne (0.5 tsp)
- Chicken thighs (8, boneless, skinless, bite-sized pieces)
- Cloves (0.5 tsp, ground)
- Garlic powder (0.75 Tbsp.)
- Ground cumin (0.75 Tbsp.)
- Lemon juice (1 lemon)
- Olive oil (0.33 c.)
- Onion (1, sliced thinly)
- Paprika (0.75 Tbsp.)
- Salt
- Turmeric powder (0.75 Tbsp.)

To serve:

- Pita pockets (6)
- Tzatziki sauce
- Arugula
- Diced tomatoes
- Diced onions
- Sliced Kalamata olives

Instructions:

1. Combine all spices. Then, place all chicken, already diced, into the bowl. Coat well, then toss in onions, lemon juice, and oil. Mix well and let marinade for at least 3 hours, or overnight.

2. Preheat the oven to 425 F. Allow chicken to sit at room temperature a few minutes. Then, spread it on an oiled sheet pan. Roast for 30 minutes.

3. To serve, fill up a pita pocket with tzatziki, chicken, arugula, and any toppings you prefer. Enjoy.

Turkey Mediterranean Casserole

Serves: 6

Time: 35 minutes

Ingredients:

- Fusilli pasta (0.5 lbs.)
- Turkey (1.5 c., chopped)
- Sun dried tomatoes (2 Tbsp., drained)
- Canned artichokes (7 oz., drained)
- Kalamata olives (3.5 oz., drained and chopped)
- Parsley (0.5 Tbsp., chopped and fresh)
- Basil (1 T, fresh)
- Salt and pepper to taste
- Marinara sauce (1 c.)

- Black chopped olives (2 oz., drained)
- Mozzarella cheese (1.5 c., shredded)

Instructions:

1. Warm your oven to 350 F. Prepare your pasta according to the directions, drain, and place into a bowl. Prepare your basil, parsley, olives, tomatoes, artichokes, and other ingredients.
2. Mix together the pasta with the turkey, tomatoes, olives, artichokes, herbs, seasoning, and marinara sauce. Give it a good mix to incorporate all of the ingredients evenly.
3. Take a 9x13 oven-safe dish and layer in the first half of your pasta mixture. Then, sprinkle on half of your mozzarella cheese. Top with the rest of the pasta, then sprinkle on the chopped black olives as well. Spread the rest of the shredded cheese on top, then bake it for 20-25 minutes. It is done when the cheese is all bubbly and the casserole is hot.

Heirloom Tomato and Cucumber Toast

Serves: 2

Time: 5 minutes

Ingredients:

- Heirloom tomato (1, diced)
- Persian cucumber (1, diced)
- Extra virgin olive oil (1 tsp)
- Oregano (a pinch, dried)
- Kosher salt and pepper
- Whipped cream cheese (2 tsp)
- Whole grain bread (2 pieces)
- Balsamic glaze (1 tsp)

Instructions:

4. Combine the tomato, cucumber, oil, and all seasonings together.
5. Spread cheese across bread, then top with mixture, followed by balsamic glaze.

Chapter 3: Maintaining Your Diet

Sticking to a diet can be tough. You could see that other people are having some great food and wish that you could enjoy it too. You might realize that you miss the foods that you used to eat and feel like it's a drag to not be able to enjoy them. When you are able to enjoy the foods that you are eating, sticking to your diet is far easier. However, that doesn't mean that you won't miss those old foods sometimes. Thankfully, the Mediterranean diet is not a very restrictive one—you are able to enjoy foods in moderation that would otherwise not be allowed, and because of that, you can take the slice of cake at the work party, or you can choose to pick up a coffee for yourself every now and then. When you do this, you're not doing anything wrong, so long as you enjoy food in moderation.

Within this chapter, we are going to take a look at several tips that you can use that will help you with maintaining your diet so that you will be able to stick to it, even when you feel like things are getting difficult. Think of this as your guide to avoiding giving in entirely—this will help you to do the best thing for yourself so that you can know that you are healthy. Now, let's get started.

Find Your Motivation

First, if you want to keep yourself on your diet, one of the best things that you can do is make sure that you find and stick to your motivation. Make sure that you know what it is in life that is motivating you. Are you losing weight because a doctor told you to? Fair enough—but how do you make that personal and about yourself? Maybe instead of looking at it as a purely health-related choice, look at it as something that you are doing because of yourself. Maybe you are eating better so that you are able to watch your children graduate or so that you can run after them at the park and stay healthy, even when it is hard to do so.

Remind Yourself Why You are Eating Healthily

When you find that you are struggling to eat healthily, remind yourself of why you are doing it in the first place. When you do this enough, you will begin to resist the urges easier than ever. Make it a point to tell yourself not to eat something a certain way. Take the time to remind yourself that you don't need to order that greasy pizza—you are eating better foods because you want to be there for your children or grandchildren.

Reminding yourself of your motivation is a great way to overcome those cravings that you may have at any point in time. The cravings that you have are usually strong and compelling, but if you learn to overcome them, you realize that they weren't actually as powerful as you thought they were. Defeat the cravings. Learn to tell yourself that they are not actually able to control you. Tell yourself that you can do better with yourself.

Eat Slowly

Now, on the Mediterranean diet, you should already be eating your meals with other people anyway. You should be taking the time to enjoy those meals while talking to other people and ensuring that you get that connection with them, and in doing so, you realize that you are able to do better. You realize that you are able to keep yourself under control longer, and that is a great way to defend and protect yourself from overeating.

When you eat slowly, you can get the same effect. Eating slowly means that you will have longer for your brain to realize that you should be eating less. When you are able to trigger that sensation of satiety because you were eating slowly, you end up eating fewer calories by default, and that matters immensely.

Keep Yourself Accountable

Don't forget that, ultimately, your diet is something that you must control on your own. Keep yourself accountable by making sure that you show other people what you are doing. If you are trying to lose weight, let them know, and tell them how you plan to do so. When you do this, you are able to remind yourself that other people know what you are doing and why—this is a great way to foster that sense of accountability because you will feel like you have to actually follow through, or you will be embarrassed by having to admit fault. You could also make accountability to yourself as well. When you do this, you are able to remind yourself that your diet is your own. Using apps to track your food and caloric intake is just one way that you can do this.

Remember Your Moderation

While it can be difficult to face a diet where you feel like you can't actually enjoy the foods that you would like to eat, the truth is that on the Mediterranean diet, you are totally okay to eat those foods that you like or miss if you do so in moderation. There is nothing that is absolutely forbidden on the Mediterranean diet—there are just foods that you should be restricting regularly. However, that doesn't mean that you can't have a treat every now and then.

Remembering to live in moderation will help you from feeling like you have to cheat or give up as well. When you are able to enjoy your diet and still enjoy the times where you want to enjoy your treats, you realize that there is actually a happy medium between sticking to the diet and deciding to quit entirely.

Identify the Difference between Hunger and Craving

Another great way to help yourself stick to your diet is to recognize that there is a very real difference between actually being hungry and just craving something to eat. In general, cravings are felt in the mouth—when you feel like you are salivating or like you need to eat something, but it is entirely in your head and mouth, you know that you have a craving. When you are truly hungry, you feel an emptiness in your stomach—you are able to know because your abdomen is where the motivation is coming from.

Being able to tell when you have a craving and when you are genuinely hungry, you can usually avoid eating extra calories that you didn't actually need. This is major—if you don't want to overeat, you need to know when your body actually needs something and when it just wants something. And if you find that you just want something, that's okay too—just find a way to move on from it. If you want to indulge a bit here and there, there's no harm in that!

Stick to the Meal Plan

When it comes to sticking to a diet, one of the easiest and most straightforward ways to do so is to just stick to your meal plan that you set up. You have it there for a reason—it is there for you to fall back on, and the sooner that you are willing to accept that, recognizing that ultimately, you can stay on track when you don't have to think about things too much, the better you will do. You will be able to succeed on your diet because you will know that you have those tools in place to protect you—they will be lined up to ensure that your diet is able to provide you with everything that you need and they will also be there so that you can know that you are on the right track.

Drink Plenty of Water

Another key to keeping yourself on track with your diet is to make sure that you drink plenty of water throughout the day. Oftentimes, we mistake our thirst with hunger and eat instead. Of course, if you're thirsty, food isn't going to really fix your problem, and you will end up continuing to mix up the sensation as you try to move past it. The more you eat, the thirstier you will get until you realize that you're full but still feeling "hungry." By drinking plenty of water any time that you think that you might want to eat, you will be able to keep yourself hydrated, and in addition, you will prevent yourself from unintentionally eating too much.

Eat Several Times Per Day

One of the best ways to keep yourself on track with your diet is to make sure that you are regularly eating. By eating throughout the day, making sure that you keep yourself full, it is easier to keep yourself strong enough to resist giving in to cravings or anything else. When you do this regularly, you will discover that you can actually keep away much of your cravings so that you are more successful in managing your diet.

Eating several times per day often involves small meals and snacks if you prefer to do so. Some people don't like doing this, but if you find that you're one of those people who will do well on a diet when you are never actually hungry enough to get desperate enough to break it, you will probably be just fine.

Fill Up on Protein

Another great way to protect yourself from giving in and caving on your diet is to make sure that you fill up on protein. Whether it comes from an animal or plant source, make sure that every time you eat, you have some sort of tangible protein source. This is the best way to keep yourself on track because protein keeps you fuller for longer. When you eat something that's loaded up with protein, you don't feel the need to eat as much later on. The protein is usually very dense, and that means that you get to resist feeling hungry for longer than you thought that you would.

Some easy proteins come from nuts—but make sure that you are mindful that you do not end up overeating during this process—you might unintentionally end up eating too many without realizing it. While you should be eating proteins regularly, make sure that you are mindful of calorie content as well!

Keep Only Healthy Foods

A common mistake that people make while dieting is that they end up caving when they realize that their home is filled up with foods that they shouldn't be eating. Perhaps you are the only person in your home that is attempting to diet. In this case, you may end up running into a situation where you have all sorts of non-compliant foods on hand. You might have chips for your kids or snacks that your partner likes to eat on hand. You may feel like it is difficult for you to stay firm when you have that to consider, and that means that you end up stuck in temptation.

One of the best ways to prevent this is to either cut all of the unhealthy junk out of your home entirely or make sure that you keep the off-limits foods in specific places so that you don't have to look at it and see it tempting you every time that you go to get a snack for yourself. By trying to keep yourself limited to just healthy foods, you will be healthier, and you will make better decisions.

Eat Breakfast Daily

Finally, make sure that breakfast is non-negotiable. Make sure that you enjoy it every single day, even if you're busy. This is where those make-ahead meals can come in handy; by knowing that you have to keep to a meal plan and knowing that you already have the food on hand, you can keep yourself fed. Breakfast sets you up for success or failure—if you want to truly succeed on your diet, you must make sure that you are willing to eat those healthier foods as much as possible, and you must get started on the right foot. Enjoy those foods first thing every day. Eat so that you are not ravenous when you finally do decide that it is time to sit down and find something to eat. Even if you just have a smoothie or something quick to eat as you go, having breakfast will help you to persevere.

PART III

Chapter 1: 5 Reasons why most people fail to get bigger

Are you training hard but cannot increase your muscle mass? Read this chapter on the 5 reasons why you are not increasing your muscle mass: you will probably discover that you are making one of these big mistakes. Do not worry, though: understanding the problem is the first step towards solving it.

1. Do you eat enough?

The problem could be easy to solve, do you eat enough? When you embark on a journey into fitness it is can happen to get caught up in exercising and skip on the nutritional aspect. I'm sure you know that 'abs are made in the kitchen'; well, it could not be truer. Eating enough calories (and good ones) is the first step towards getting leaner.

To increase your muscle mass, you have to eat the right amount of the right food, including carbohydrates, proteins, and fats. Your body uses the food you eat to build new muscle tissue after you destroyed the old one in training. In order to do that, it is important to consume enough protein.

Some of the best sources of protein are:

- Chicken
- Fish
- Turkey
- Lean minced meat
- eggs
- meat, broccoli, salmon

Other sources of protein

- Milk flakes
- Greek yogurt
- Quark cheese
- Beans and legumes
- Nuts

A high-protein diet is fundamental to build muscles. Experts and pro bodybuilders have stated, over the years, that consuming 1.2 – 2.0g of protein per kg of weight is a good ratio to keep building lean muscle mass over time. If you are not able to get this amount trough diet alone than food supplements can come handy

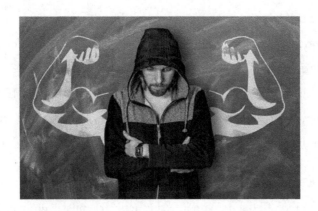

2. Do you train hard enough?

If you have been training for a while, but have not made some gains, it could be due to a lack of training. Do you train hard enough? Our body reacts quickly under pressure and if you're not increasing weights over time, then you could run into a stall zone. So do not settle!

Your body is not made to change itself and it is your duty to give it the right stimulus so that it can actually grow. If you want to get faster results, add more intensity to your training.

3.   Rest and recovery

Rest is a fundamental aspect when it comes to any fitness routine. Your muscles require rest to grow stronger and that is the reason why so many athletes choose a training routine divided into days. For example, one day they train legs and the day after the arms, making sure that every part of the body receives at least one day of rest (try to train every muscle group at least once a week).

Even sleeping is very important: when we sleep deeply our bodies repair muscle fibres. It is recommended to sleep 8 hours per night, although my advice is to sleep more if you can.

4.   Do you drink too much alcohol?

Drinking too much alcohol can destroy muscle growth. Alcohol does not contain valuable nutrients but has many calories, 7 per gram to be precise. As a result, it is easy to "drink your calories" without even thinking about it. If you are on a fitness regimen of any kind, it is advisable to avoid alcohol consumption. However, a drink has never killed anybody, just be reasonable.

5.   Are you over-training?

Training with high frequency and intensity activates muscle growth. Therefore, it is fundamental to train different days during the week: 4 days of weight training and 1-2 of aerobic activity is advisable. If you begin a program, complete it! Too many times athletes give up or say that a certain workout does not work "for them" (as if this could be a thing), but the key is constancy. It may take a while to see results, do not give up!

Many bodybuilders, like Arnold, have mentioned the famous 'mind and body connection', so try to keep your attention on the muscle you are training while you do the exercises. It is also a question of 'sensations' and how your muscles contract and expand.

Instead of simply doing the training, focus on the exercise and visualize the growth you are generating.

Chapter 2: 10 Rules to increase your muscle mass

It is always challenging to give the 10 rules of anything. However, when it comes to growing muscles, it is important to have some guidance. This is why we give you 10 rules to increase your lean muscle mass for a more defined body.

1. Give space to recovery: it is not true that more is better, especially for the frequency. It is true that you can train only 1 muscle a day and then before you go back to training that muscle should pass 6/8 days, but the organs of "disposal" are always the same and run the risk of overloading. You can make short periods with high frequency, but these must then have periods of supercompensation.

2. You should sleep very well: it is not only the quantity (7/9 hours per night) but the quality of sleep. An excellent component of deep sleep, it is the basic element for recovery and growth. Sleep must be mainly nocturnal, it is well known by those who work for shifts that daytime sleep has different qualities.

3. Eat often: at least 6 times, breakfast, mid-morning, lunch, afternoon, dinner and after dinner; and in any case, use the rule of about 2.5 hours between one meal and another. If you spend many hours between lunch and dinner, introduce two snacks in the afternoon.

4. Eat a balanced diet: with every meal, give space to all the nutrients. Not only proteins and carbohydrates, fats are also great allies, since are hormonal mediators, provide calories and improve recovery.

5. Do not train too long: do not spend too much time working on your endurance, since it does more harm than good to muscle's growth.

6. Think positive: the mind is a great ally for the optimization of metabolic processes; Positivity helps the hormonal systems to overcome the

negativity generated by the inevitable obstacles and setbacks of everyday life. It is essential to define the goals (even in the short term) to go to the gym with clear ideas already, aware that you will have an excellent training session.

7. Rely on basic movements: squats, deadlifts, bench, lunges, are the fundamentals; mass is not built by abusing side wings, crosses or arms. Dedicate yourself to these exercises by changing sets, repetitions and recovery times. Then there may be periods in which the complementary serve to unload the joints and give a different kind of intensity.

8. Do not just focus on some muscle groups: first, you have to build a solid foundation, do not do like those beginners who already after 6 months want to focus only on one or two muscles.

9. Use the right supplements: pay attention, do not abuse them, simply select the main ones; good proteins, BCAAs (branched amino acids) or a pool of amino acids, glutamine, creatine, a support for your joints, HMB. These are already more than enough to support and integrate a diet that must follow the correct guidelines.

10. Choose a motivating gym: well-equipped but with what you really need, lots of dumbbells and barbells, benches and maybe 2 racks for the squat. Usually, in these environments, you can also find training partners to share workouts, goals and discussions. Training in a sterile and "losing" environment is certainly not very motivating and does not establish the spirit necessary to achieve the goals.

The points to be developed would still be many but in reality, with the 10 you have read you are already well on your way to get bigger and leaner. Success is built from the basics, especially when you are just starting out.

Chapter 3: How to actually build lean muscles

It is difficult to build muscle mass, but with constancy you can do it; however, if you want to develop it quickly, you can find some compromises, like accept to gain some fat along with muscle mass and stop some other type of training, such as running, so that the body starts to focus on developing muscles. You also need to eat more by using the right strategies and doing those physical activities that allow you to increase your muscles. Here are some of the key steps to build lean muscles for real.

1. Start with a basic strength training. Most of the exercises that involve the main muscle groups start with a strength training that activates more joints and that allows you to lift a whole greater weight, such as bench presses for the pectorals, those behind the head for the deltoids, the rower with a barbell for the back and the squats for the legs. They are all exercises that allow you to lift heavier weights while still remaining active and keeping enough energy to better stimulate muscle growth.

2. Engaged thoroughly. The key to developing muscle mass is to do high intensity exercises; with a light exercise, even if protracted in time, the muscles almost never find the right conditions for decomposition and then rebuild. Schedule sessions for 30-45 minutes 3-4 times a week (every other day); it may seem like an easily manageable schedule but remember that during each session you have to engage as intensely as possible. Initially, the muscles may be sore, but over time the routine will become easier.

3. During each training session, only lift the weights that you are able to support by assuming the correct posture. Test your limits to find the right ballast you can lift, doing different repetitions with different dumbbells. You should be able to do 3-4 sets of 8-12 repetitions without feeling the

need to put them on the ground; if you are not able, reduce the weights. In general, 6-12 repetitions stimulate the growth of the volume of the muscles, while fewer repetitions favour the increase of the strength at the expense of the size of the same. If you can do 10 or more repetitions without experiencing a burning sensation, you can increase the weight; remember that you do not increase muscle mass until you challenge yourself to the limit.

4. Lift weights explosively. Raise the handlebars quickly but lower them slowly.

5. Keep the correct posture. To develop a precise technique, you have to do each repetition in the right way; beginners must commit to doing only the repetitions that they are able to perform based on the level of resistance. Find your rhythm for each exercise; you do not have to reach muscle failure when you're at the beginning. You should be able to complete the whole movement without getting to bend down or change position; if you cannot, switch to less heavy dumbbells. In most cases, it starts with the arms or legs extended. During the first sets, you should work with a personal trainer who will teach you the correct posture of the various exercises before continuing alone.

6. Toggle the muscle groups. You do not have to keep the same group moving at every set, otherwise, you may get to damage your muscles, so be sure to alternate, so every time you train you can work intensely for an hour on a different muscle group. If you do physical activity three times a week, try doing the exercises as follows:

First session: do exercises for the chest, triceps and biceps;

Second session: concentrate on the legs;

Third session: do abs and chest

7. Be careful not to reach a stall level. If you always do the same exercise repeatedly, you cannot get improvements; you have to increase the weight of the barbell and when you reach a plateau even with this, change exercise. Be aware of progress and see if your muscles do not seem to change, because it may be a sign that you need to make changes in your physical activity routine.

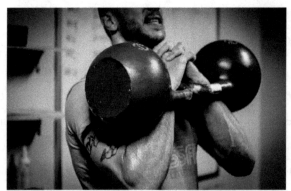

8. Rest between one workout and another. For those who have a rapid metabolism, the rest period is almost as important as the exercise itself. The body needs time to regenerate muscle mass without burning too many calories by doing other activities. Running and other cardio exercises can effectively prevent muscle growth; then take a break between the different sessions. Sleep well at night, so that you feel regenerated for the next session.

9. Create a mind/muscle connection. Some research has found that it can optimize results in the gym. Instead of focusing on your day or the girl next to you, committed to developing a muscle-oriented mindset that helps you achieve your goals. Here's how:

Every time you complete a repetition, visualize the muscle growth you wish to achieve.

If you are lifting with one hand, place the other on the muscle you wish to develop; in this way, you should perceive exactly which muscle fibres are working and you can stay focused on the effort.

Remember that the amount of weight on the bar is not as important as you may think, but it is the effect that weight has on the muscle that allows you to get the volume and strength you are looking for; this process is closely related to the mentality and the goal of your concentration.

10. Eat whole foods rich in calories. You should get the calories from nutritious whole foods, so you have the right energy to quickly accumulate muscle mass. Those rich in sugar, white flour, trans fats and added flavours contain many calories but few nutrients and increase the fat instead of developing the muscle. If you want to develop the muscles and their definition, you have to opt for a wide variety of whole foods that are part of all the food groups.

11. Eat protein rich in calories, like steak and roast beef, roast chicken (with skin and dark meat), salmon, eggs and pork; proteins are essential when you want to increase muscle mass. Avoid bacon, sausages and other sausages, because they contain additives that are not suitable if you eat it in large quantities.

12. Consume lots of fruit and vegetables of all kinds; these foods provide the essential fiber and nutrients, as well as keeping you well hydrated.

13. Do not neglect whole grains, such as oatmeal, whole wheat, buckwheat and quinoa; avoid white bread, biscuits, muffins, pancakes, waffles and other similar foods.

14. Add legumes and nuts, such as black beans, Pinto, Lima, walnuts, pecans, peanuts and almonds to your diet.

15. Eat more than you think you need. Eat when you're hungry and stop

when you feel satisfied? This may seem completely normal, but when you're trying to gain muscle mass quickly, you have to eat more than usual. Add another portion to each meal or even more if you can handle it; the body needs the energy to develop the muscles: it is a simple concept.

To this end, a good breakfast includes a cup of oatmeal, four eggs, two or more slices of grilled ham, an apple, an orange and a banana.

For lunch, you can eat a wholemeal sandwich with chicken, several handfuls of dried fruit, two avocados and a large salad of cabbage and tomatoes.

For dinner, you can consider a large steak or some other source of protein, potatoes, vegetables and double the portions of each dish.

16. Eat at least five meals a day. You must not wait to be hungry before eating again; you have to constantly replenish your body when you are trying to develop muscle mass. It will not be this way forever, so take advantage and enjoy the moment! Eat two more meals in addition to the traditional three (breakfast, lunch and dinner).

17. Take supplements, but do not solely on them. You do not have to think that protein shakes do all the work for you; for your purpose, you need to get the most calories from high-calorie whole foods; Having said that, you can definitely speed up the process by taking certain supplements that have not proven to be harmful to the body.

Creatine is a protein supplement that can increase muscle; usually, it is sold as a powder that is dissolved in water and drunk a few times a day.

Protein shakes are fine when you cannot get enough calories through normal meals.

18. Keep yourself hydrated. Training hard to gain muscle mass can quickly

dehydrate you. To cope with this risk, always carry a bottle of water with you wherever you go and drink whenever you are thirsty; in theory, you should drink about 3 litres of fluids a day, but you should drink more, especially before and after training.

Avoid sugary or carbonated drinks, because they do not help your overall fitness and may even take you back when you do strength exercises.

Alcohol is also harmful for your purpose: it dehydrates and leaves a feeling of exhaustion.

19. Try to get to know your body better. Do you know which foods are effective for you and which are not? During this phase of change, pay attention to what happens to your muscles. Each person is different and the food that is not suitable for one person can instead be very useful for another; if you do not notice improvements within a week, make changes and try something else the following week.

20. Sleep more than what you think you should. Sleep is essential to allow muscles to develop; try to sleep at least seven hours a night, although the ideal would be 8-9 hours.

21. Focus only on strength training. You may like to do cardio exercises (sports like running and so on), but these activities require a further effort of the body (muscles and joints) and consume the energy you need to build muscle mass. In general, cardio activities should be included in an exercise routine for general health and well-being, but if you are currently struggling to increase muscle volume quickly, you need to focus on this for a few months, so you can reach your goal.

Chapter 4: Tips to keep making gains

- Always ask a friend for help when doing the most difficult lifting exercises, such as bench press; these are high risk movements and it is always important to have some support to be able to do more repetitions.

- Keep motivation high. Find a friend who's training with you, sign up for a weightlifting fan forum or keep a diary to monitor progress; whatever you choose, the important thing is that you inspire yourself.

- If you currently do not have dumbbells and you've never done weight lifting so far, start with push-ups and chin-ups, which are quite challenging for a beginner.

- Make the push-ups easier: start from the normal position of the push-ups and lower the body very slowly; go down as far as possible without touching the floor with your chest and abs. Later, relieved after resting your knees on the ground and start again. This is an excellent solution when you are not yet strong enough to be able to do traditional push-ups.

- Make sure you stay focused. Take breaks only when you need them and not when you feel tired; it is only in this way that you can develop psychological endurance.

Chapter 5: Example of a training schedule

The frequency of this hypothetical schedule for mass training, provides 4 days of training per week, with about 10-12 repetitions per exercise.

The mass program is a middle ground between heavy weights / high intensity training and volume/pump training. You work on strength, hypertrophy, rotating muscle definition and progression, accustoming the body to weight and intensity of work with a growing load plan, which reaches your ideal combination for mass growth.

It is essential, in fact, to know your body and your own ceilings, to prepare and act upon a successful program.

Weekly training schedule (Monday - Friday)

Chest and abs

Legs

Rest

Shoulders - triceps

Back - biceps

Daily mass gym program

1st day - chest and abs

Crossed exercises with dumbbells - flat bench

Distances with barbell - flat bench

Multipower inclined (or with dumbbells)

Cross exercises with cables

Crunches (3 sets - 15 repetitions)

Abs with elbows in support and knees on the chest (3 sets - 15 repetitions)

2nd Day - legs

45-degree press

Squat with barbell

Standing calf (3 sets - 15 repetitions)

Seated calf (3 sets - 15 repetitions)

Leg extension

Leg curl

3rd Day - shoulders and deltoids

Slow forward exercise with barbell - seated

Pull at the bottom with a barbell

Lateral raises with dumbbells

Push down

French press around the neck with a barbell

Bench presses

4th Day - back

Pull ups

Pullover

Pulley

Deadlift

Curl with dumbbells

Curl reverse socket with a barbell

Recovery between the series should be carried out for about 1 minute and a half (1 '30).

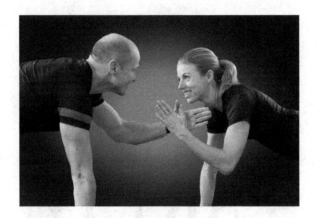

The first month these exercises should be performed with at least 3 sets and about 10-12 repetitions, with non-high loads. In case you are not trained enough, you can think of sets of 12-10-8 repetitions, where you start with 12 and perform 8 repetitions in the third set.

The second month you can go up to 4 sets with 10 repetitions or 12 if the body keeps up with the pace. It will not be easy to get to the twelfth repetition without fatigue and, in this case, you can also think about dropping with weights and get to 12 repetitions with lighter loads.

The third month you have to keep the pace but without progressing too much, with the initials 3 sets of 12 repetitions per exercise.

PART IV

Smoothie Diet Recipes

The smoothie diet is all about replacing some of your meals with smoothies that are loaded with veggies and fruits. It has been found that the smoothie diet is very helpful in losing weight along with excess fat. The ingredients of the smoothies will vary, but they will focus mainly on vegetables and fruits. The best part about the smoothie diet is that there is no need to count your calorie intake and less food tracking. The diet is very low in calories and is also loaded with phytonutrients.

Apart from weight loss, there are various other benefits of the smoothie diet. It can help you to stay full for a longer time as most smoothies are rich in fiber. It can also help you to control your cravings as smoothies are full of flavor and nutrients. Whenever you feel like snacking, just prepare a smoothie, and you are good to go. Also, smoothies can aid in digestion as they are rich in important minerals and vitamins. Fruits such as mango are rich in carotenoids that can help in improving your skin quality. As the smoothie diet is mainly based on veggies and fruits, it can detoxify your body.

In this section, you will find various recipes of smoothies that you can include in your smoothie diet.

Chapter 1: Fruit Smoothies

The best way of having fruits is by making smoothies. Fruit smoothies can help you start your day with loads of nutrients so that you can remain energetic throughout the day. Here are some easy-to-make fruit smoothie recipes that you can enjoy during any time of the day.

Quick Fruit Smoothie

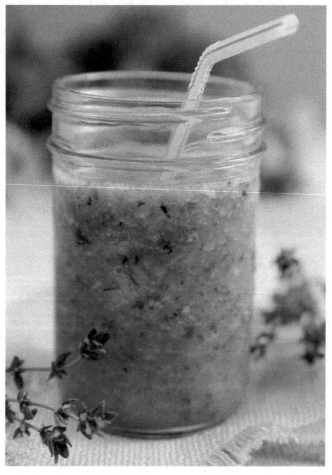

Total Prep & Cooking Time: Fifteen minutes

Yields: Four servings

Nutrition Facts: Calories: 115.2 | Protein: 1.2g | Carbs: 27.2g | Fat: 0.5g | Fiber: 3.6g

Ingredients

- One cup of strawberries
- One banana (cut in chunks)
- Two peaches
- Two cups of ice
- One cup of orange and mango juice

Method:

1. Add banana, strawberries, and peaches in a blender.

2. Blend until frothy and smooth.

3. Add the orange and mango juice and blend again. Add ice for adjusting the consistency and blend for two minutes.

4. Divide the smoothie in glasses and serve with mango chunks from the top.

Triple Threat Smoothie

Total Prep & Cooking Time: Ten minutes

Yields: Four servings

Nutrition Facts: Calories: 132.2 | Protein: 3.4g | Carbs: 27.6g | Fat: 1.3g | Fiber: 2.7g

Ingredients

- One kiwi (sliced)
- One banana (chopped)
- One cup of each
    - Ice cubes
    - Strawberries
- Half cup of blueberries
- One-third cup of orange juice
- Eight ounces of peach yogurt

Method:

1. Add kiwi, strawberries, and bananas in a food processor.

2. Blend until smooth.

3. Add the blueberries along with orange juice. Blend again for two minutes.

4. Add peach yogurt and ice cubes. Give it a pulse.

5. Pour the prepared smoothie in smoothie glasses and serve with blueberry chunks from the top.

Tropical Smoothie

Total Prep & Cooking Time: Fifteen minutes

Yields: Two servings

Nutrition Facts: Calories: 127.3 | Protein: 1.6g | Carbs: 30.5g | Fat: 0.7g | Fiber: 4.2g

Ingredients

- One mango (seeded)
- One papaya (cubed)
- Half cup of strawberries
- One-third cup of orange juice
- Five ice cubes

Method:

1. Add mango, strawberries, and papaya in a blender. Blend the ingredients until smooth.

2. Add ice cubes and orange juice for adjusting the consistency.

3. Blend again.

4. Serve with strawberry chunks from the top.

Fruit and Mint Smoothie

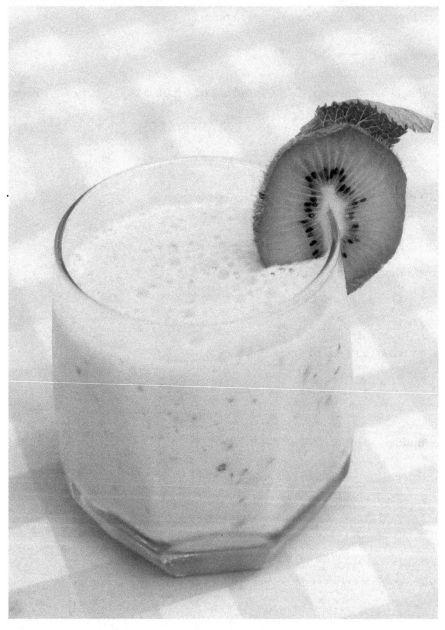

Total Prep & Cooking Time: Fifteen minutes

Yields: Two servings

Nutrition Facts: Calories: 90.3 | Protein: 0.7g | Carbs: 21.4g | Fat: 0.4g | Fiber: 2.5g

Ingredients

- One-fourth cup of each
    - Applesauce (unsweetened)
    - Red grapes (seedless, frozen)
- One tbsp. of lime juice
- Three strawberries (frozen)
- One cup of pineapple cubes
- Three mint leaves

Method:

1. Add grapes, lime juice, and applesauce in a blender. Blend the ingredients until frothy and smooth.

2. Add pineapple cubes, mint leaves, and frozen strawberries in the blender. Pulse the ingredients for a few times until the pineapple and strawberries are crushed.

3. Serve with mint leaves from the top.

Banana Smoothie

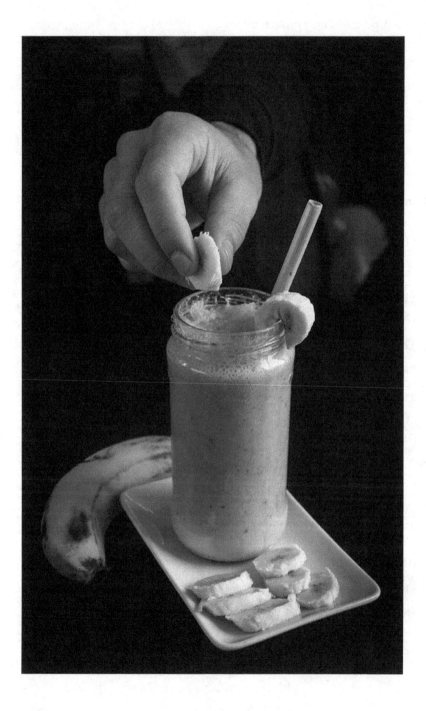

Total Prep & Cooking Time: Ten minutes

Yields: Four servings

Nutrition Facts: Calories: 122.6 | Protein: 1.3g | Carbs: 34.6g | Fat: 0.4g | Fiber: 2.2g

Ingredients

- Three bananas (sliced)
- One cup of fresh pineapple juice
- One tbsp. of honey
- Eight cubes of ice

Method:

1. Combine the bananas and pineapple juice in a blender.

2. Blend until smooth.

3. Add ice cubes along with honey.

4. Blend for two minutes.

5. Serve immediately.

Dragon Fruit Smoothie

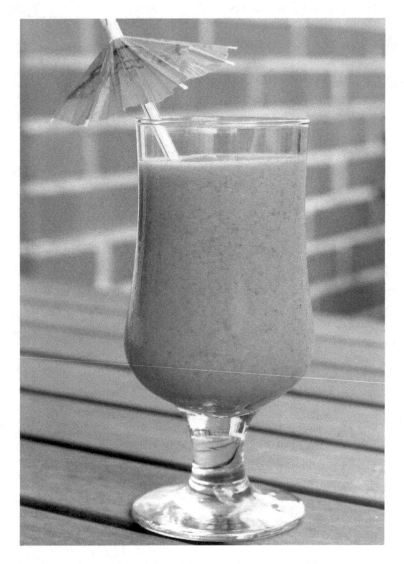

Total Prep & Cooking Time: Twenty minutes

Yields: Four servings

Nutrition Facts: Calories: 147.6 | Protein: 5.2g | Carbs: 21.4g | Fat: 6.4g | Fiber: 2.9g

Ingredients

- One-fourth cup of almonds
- Two tbsps. of shredded coconut
- One tsp. of chocolate chips
- One cup of yogurt
- One dragon fruit (chopped)
- Half cup of pineapple cubes
- One tbsp. of honey

Method:

1. Add almonds, dragon fruit, coconut, and chocolate chips in a high power blender. Blend until smooth.

2. Add yogurt, pineapple, and honey. Blend well.

3. Serve with chunks of dragon fruit from the top.

Kefir Blueberry Smoothie

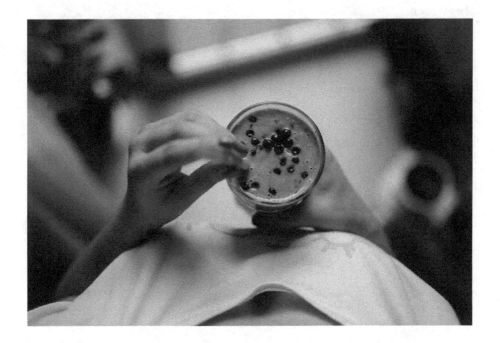

Total Prep & Cooking Time: Fifteen minutes

Yields: Two servings

Nutrition Facts: Calories: 304.2 | Protein: 7.3g | Carbs: 41.3g | Fat: 13.2g | Fiber: 4.6g

Ingredients

- Half cup of kefir
- One cup of blueberries (frozen)
- Half banana (cubed)

- One tbsp. of almond butter
- Two tsps. of honey

Method:

1. Add blueberries, banana cubes, and kefir in a blender.

2. Blend until smooth.

3. Add honey and almond butter.

4. Pulse the smoothie for a few times.

5. Serve immediately.

Ginger Fruit Smoothie

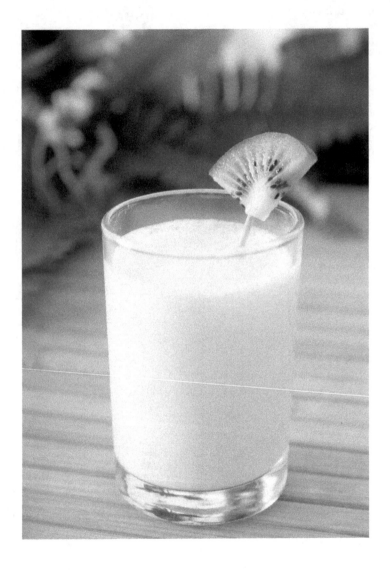

Total Prep & Cooking Time: Fifteen minutes

Yields: Two servings

Nutrition Facts: Calories: 160.2 | Protein: 1.9g | Carbs: 41.3g | Fat: 0.7g | Fiber: 5.6g

Ingredients

- One-fourth cup of each
    - Blueberries (frozen)
    - Green grapes (seedless)
- Half cup of green apple (chopped)
- One cup of water
- Three strawberries
- One piece of ginger
- One tbsp. of agave nectar

Method:

1. Add blueberries, grapes, and water in a blender. Blend the ingredients.

2. Add green apple, strawberries, agave nectar, and ginger. Blend for making thick slushy.

3. Serve immediately.

Fruit Batido

Total Prep & Cooking Time: Fifteen minutes

Yields: Six servings

Nutrition Facts: Calories: 129.3 | Protein: 4.2g | Carbs: 17.6g | Fat: 4.6g | Fiber: 0.6g

Ingredients

- One can of evaporated milk
- One cup of papaya (chopped)
- One-fourth cup of white sugar
- One tsp. of vanilla extract
- One tsp. of cinnamon (ground)
- One tray of ice cubes

Method:

1. Add papaya, white sugar, cinnamon, and vanilla extract in a food processor. Blend the ingredients until smooth.

2. Add milk and ice cubes. Blend for making slushy.

3. Serve immediately.

Banana Peanut Butter Smoothie

Total Prep & Cooking Time: Ten minutes

Yields: Four servings

Nutrition Facts: Calories: 332 | Protein: 13.2g | Carbs: 35.3g | Fat: 17.8g | Fiber: 3.9g

Ingredients

- Two bananas (cubed)
- Two cups of milk
- Half cup of peanut butter
- Two tbsps. of honey
- Two cups of ice cubes

Method:

1. Add banana cubes and peanut butter in a blender. Blend for making a smooth paste.

2. Add milk, ice cubes, and honey. Blend the ingredients until smooth.

3. Serve with banana chunks from the top.

Chapter 2: Breakfast Smoothies

Smoothie forms an essential part of breakfast in the smoothie diet plan. Here are some breakfast smoothie recipes for you that can be included in your daily breakfast plan.

Berry Banana Smoothie

Total Prep & Cooking Time: Twenty minutes

Yields: Two servings

Nutrition Facts: Calories: 330 | Protein: 6.7g | Carbs: 56.3g | Fat: 13.2g | Fiber: 5.5g

Ingredients

- One cup of each
  - Strawberries
  - Peaches (cubed)
  - Apples (cubed)
- One banana (cubed)
- Two cups of vanilla ice cream
- Half cup of ice cubes
- One-third cup of milk

Method:

1. Place strawberries, peaches, banana, and apples in a blender. Pulse the ingredients.

2. Add milk, ice cream, and ice cubes. Blend the smoothie until frothy and smooth.

3. Serve with a scoop of ice cream from the top.

Berry Surprise

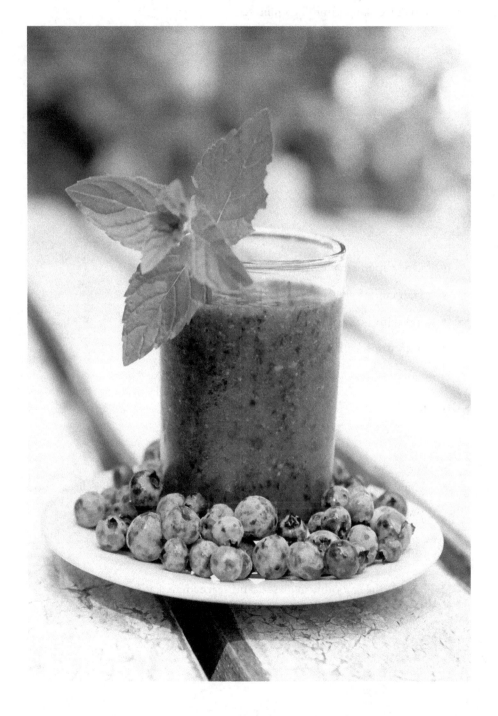

Total Prep & Cooking Time: Ten minutes

Yields: Two servings

Nutrition Facts: Calories: 164.2 | Protein: 1.2g | Carbs: 40.2g | Fat: 0.4g | Fiber: 4.8g

Ingredients

- One cup of strawberries
- Half cup of pineapple cubes
- One-third cup of raspberries
- Two tbsps. of limeade concentrate (frozen)

Method:

1. Combine pineapple cubes, strawberries, and raspberries in a food processor. Blend the ingredients until smooth.

2. Add the frozen limeade and blend again.

3. Divide the smoothie in glasses and serve immediately.

Coconut Matcha Smoothie

Total Prep & Cooking Time: Twenty minutes

Yields: Two servings

Nutrition Facts: Calories: 362 | Protein: 7.2g | Carbs: 70.1g | Fat: 8.7g | Fiber: 12.1g

Ingredients

- One large banana
- One cup of frozen mango cubes
- Two leaves of kale (torn)
- Three tbsps. of white beans (drained)
- Two tbsps. of shredded coconut (unsweetened)
- Half tsp. of matcha green tea (powder)
- Half cup of water

Method:

1. Add cubes of mango, banana, white beans, and kale in a blender. Blend all the ingredients until frothy and smooth.

2. Add shredded coconut, white beans, water, and green tea powder. Blend for thirty seconds.

3. Serve with shredded coconut from the top.

Cantaloupe Frenzy

Total Prep & Cooking Time: Ten minutes

Yields: Three servings

Nutrition Facts: Calories: 108.3 | Protein: 1.6g | Carbs: 26.2g | Fat: 0.2g | Fiber: 1.6g

Ingredients

- One cantaloupe (seeded, chopped)
- Three tbsps. of white sugar
- Two cups of ice cubes

Method:

1. Place the chopped cantaloupe along with white sugar in a blender. Puree the mixture.

2. Add cubes of ice and blend again.

3. Pour the smoothie in serving glasses. Serve immediately.

Berry Lemon Smoothie

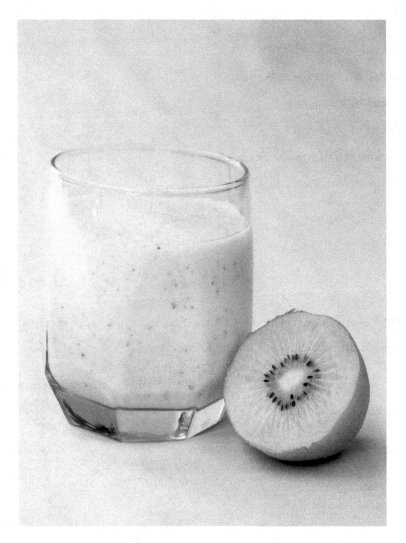

Total Prep & Cooking Time: Ten minutes

Yields: Four servings

Nutrition Facts: Calories: 97.2 | Protein: 5.4g | Carbs: 19.4g | Fat: 0.4g | Fiber: 1.8g

Ingredients

- Eight ounces of blueberry yogurt
- One and a half cup of milk (skim)
- One cup of ice cubes
- Half cup of blueberries
- One-third cup of strawberries
- One tsp. of lemonade mix

Method:

1. Add blueberry yogurt, skim milk, blueberries, and strawberries in a food processor. Blend the ingredients until smooth.

2. Add lemonade mix and ice cubes. Pulse the mixture for making a creamy and smooth smoothie.

3. Divide the smoothie in glasses and serve.

Orange Glorious

Total Prep & Cooking Time: Ten minutes

Yields: Four servings

Nutrition Facts: Calories: 212 | Protein: 3.4g | Carbs: 47.3g | Fat: 1.5g | Fiber: 0.5g

Ingredients

- Six ounces of orange juice concentrate (frozen)
- One cup of each
  - Water
  - Milk
- Half cup of white sugar
- Twelve ice cubes
- One tsp. of vanilla extract

Method:

1. Combine orange juice concentrate, white sugar, milk, and water in a blender.

2. Add vanilla extract and ice cubes. Blend the mixture until smooth.

3. Pour the smoothie in glasses and enjoy!

Grapefruit Smoothie

Total Prep & Cooking Time: Ten minutes

Yields: Two servings

Nutrition Facts: Calories: 200.3 | Protein: 4.7g | Carbs: 46.3g | Fat: 1.2g | Fiber: 7.6g

Ingredients

- Three grapefruits (peeled)
- One cup of water
- Three ounces of spinach
- Six ice cubes
- Half-inch piece of ginger
- One tsp. of flax seeds

Method:

1. Combine spinach, grapefruit, and ginger in a high power blender. Blend until smooth.

2. Add water, flax seeds, and ice cubes. Blend smooth.

3. Pour the smoothie in glasses and serve.

Sour Smoothie

Total Prep & Cooking Time: Ten minutes

Yields: Two servings

Nutrition Facts: Calories: 102.6 | Protein: 2.3g | Carbs: 30.2g | Fat: 0.7g | Fiber: 7.9g

Ingredients

- One cup of ice cubes
- Two fruit limes (peeled)
- One orange (peeled)
- One lemon (peeled)
- One kiwi (peeled)
- One tsp. of honey

Method:

1. Add fruit limes, lemon, orange, and kiwi in a food processor. Blend until frothy and smooth.

2. Add cubes of ice and honey. Pulse the ingredients.

3. Divide the smoothie in glasses and enjoy!

Ginger Orange Smoothie

Total Prep & Cooking Time: Ten minutes

Yields: One serving

Nutrition Facts: Calories: 115.6 | Protein: 2.2g | Carbs: 27.6g | Fat: 1.3g | Fiber: 5.7g

Ingredients

- One large orange
- Two carrots (peeled, cut in chunks)
- Half cup of each
  - Red grapes
  - Ice cubes
- One-fourth cup of water
- One-inch piece of ginger

Method:

1. Combine carrots, grapes, and orange in a high power blender. Blend until frothy and smooth.

2. Add ice cubes, ginger, and water. Blend the ingredients for thirty seconds.

3. Serve immediately.

Cranberry Smoothie

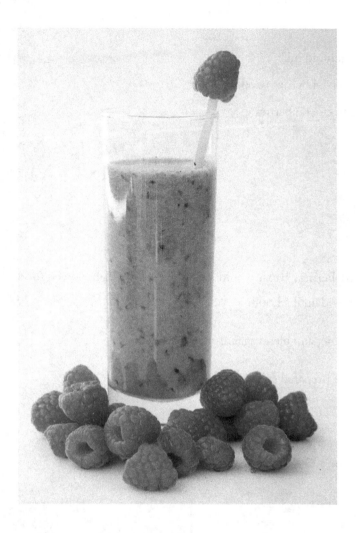

Total Prep & Cooking Time: One hour and ten minutes

Yields: Two servings

Nutrition Facts: Calories: 155.9 | Protein: 2.2g | Carbs: 33.8g | Fat: 1.6g | Fiber: 5.2g

Ingredients

- One cup of almond milk
- Half cup of mixed berries (frozen)
- One-third cup of cranberries
- One banana

Method:

1. Blend mixed berries, banana, and cranberries in a high power food processor. Blend until smooth.

2. Add almond milk and blend again for twenty seconds.

3. Refrigerate the prepared smoothie for one hour.

4. Serve chilled.

Creamsicle Smoothie

Total Prep & Cooking Time: Ten minutes

Yields: Two servings

Nutrition Facts: Calories: 121.3 | Protein: 4.7g | Carbs: 19.8g | Fat: 2.5g | Fiber: 0.3g

Ingredients

- One cup of orange juice
- One and a half cup of crushed ice
- Half cup of milk
- One tsp. of white sugar

Method:

1. Blend milk, orange juice, white sugar, and ice in a high power blender.

2. Keep blending until there is no large chunk of ice. Try to keep the consistency of slushy.

3. Serve immediately.

Sunshine Smoothie

Total Prep & Cooking Time: Thirty minutes

Yields: Four servings

Nutrition Facts: Calories: 176.8 | Protein: 4.2g | Carbs: 39.9g | Fat: 1.3g | Fiber: 3.9g

Ingredients

- Two nectarines (pitted, quartered)
- One banana (cut in chunks)
- One orange (peeled, quartered)
- One cup of vanilla yogurt
- One-third cup of orange juice
- One tbsp. of honey

Method:

1. Add banana chunks, nectarines, and orange in a blender. Blender for two minutes.

2. Add vanilla yogurt, honey, and orange juice. Blend the ingredients until frothy and smooth.

3. Pour the smoothie in glasses and serve.

Chapter 3: Vegetable Smoothies

Apart from fruit smoothies, vegetable smoothies can also provide you with essential nutrients. In fact, vegetable smoothies are tasty as well. So, here are some vegetable smoothie recipes for you.

Mango Kale Berry Smoothie
Total Prep & Cooking Time: Ten minutes

Yields: Four servings

Nutrition Facts: Calories: 117.3 | Protein: 3.1g | Carbs: 22.6g | Fat: 3.6g | Fiber: 6.2g

Ingredients

- One cup of orange juice
- One-third cup of kale
- One and a half cup of mixed berries (frozen)
- Half cup of mango chunks
- One-fourth cup of water
- Two tbsps. of chia seeds

Method:

1. Take a high power blender and add kale, orange juice, berries, mango chunks, chia seeds, and half a cup of water.

2. Blend the ingredients on high settings until smooth.

3. In case the smoothie is very thick, you can adjust the consistency by adding more water.

4. Pour the smoothie in glasses and serve.

Breakfast Pink Smoothie

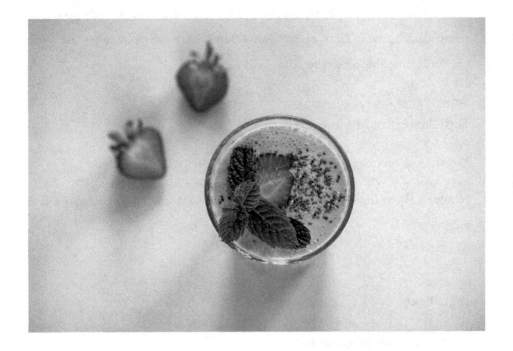

Total Prep & Cooking Time: Ten minutes

Yields: Two servings

Nutrition Facts: Calories: 198.3 | Protein: 12.3g | Carbs: 6.3g | Fat: 4.5g | Fiber: 8.8g

Ingredients

- One and a half cup of strawberries (frozen)
- One cup of raspberries
- One orange (peeled)

- Two carrots
- Two cups of coconut milk (light)
- One small beet (quartered)

Method:

1. Add strawberries, raspberries, and orange in a blender. Blend until frothy and smooth.

2. Add beet, carrots, and coconut milk.

3. Blend again for one minute.

4. Divide the smoothie in glasses and serve.

Butternut Squash Smoothie

Total Prep & Cooking Time: Five minutes

Yields: Four servings

Nutrition Facts: Calories: 127.3 | Protein: 2.3g | Carbs: 32.1g | Fat: 1.2g | Fiber: 0.6g

Ingredients

- Two cups of almond milk
- One-fourth cup of nut butter (of your choice)
- One cup of water
- One and a half cup of butternut squash (frozen)
- Two ripe bananas
- One tsp. of cinnamon (ground)
- Two tbsps. of hemp protein
- Half cup of strawberries
- One tbsp. of chia seeds
- Half tbsp. of bee pollen

Method:

1. Add butternut squash, bananas, strawberries, and almond milk in a blender. Blend until frothy and smooth.

2. Add water, nut butter, cinnamon, hemp protein, chia seeds, and bee pollen. Blend the ingredients f0r two minutes.

3. Divide the smoothie in glasses and enjoy!

Zucchini and Wild Blueberry Smoothie

Total Prep & Cooking Time: Ten minutes

Yields: Three servings

Nutrition Facts: Calories: 190.2 | Protein: 7.3g | Carbs: 27.6g | Fat: 8.1g | Fiber: 5.7g

Ingredients

- One banana
- One cup of wild blueberries (frozen)
- One-fourth cup of peas (frozen)
- Half cup of zucchini (frozen, chopped)
- One tbsp. of each
  - Hemp hearts
  - Chia seeds
  - Bee pollen
- One-third cup of almond milk
- Two tbsps. of nut butter (of your choice)
- Ten cubes of ice

Method:

1. Add blueberries, banana, peas, and zucchini in a high power blender. Blend the ingredients for two minutes.

2. Add chia seeds, hemp hearts, almond milk, bee pollen, nut butter, and ice. Blend the mixture for making a thick and smooth smoothie.

3. Pour the smoothie in glasses and serve with chopped blueberries from the top.

Cauliflower and Blueberry Smoothie

Total Prep & Cooking Time: Five minutes

Yields: Two servings

Nutrition Facts: Calories: 201.9 | Protein: 7.1g | Carbs: 32.9g | Fat: 10.3g | Fiber: 4.6g

Ingredients

- One Clementine (peeled)
- Three-fourth cup of cauliflower (frozen)
- Half cup of wild blueberries (frozen)
- One cup of Greek yogurt
- One tbsp. of peanut butter
- Bunch of spinach

Method:

1. Add cauliflower, Clementine, and blueberries in a blender. Blend for one minute.

2. Add peanut butter, spinach, and yogurt. Pulse the ingredients for two minutes until smooth.

3. Divide the prepared smoothie in glasses and enjoy!

Immunity Booster Smoothie

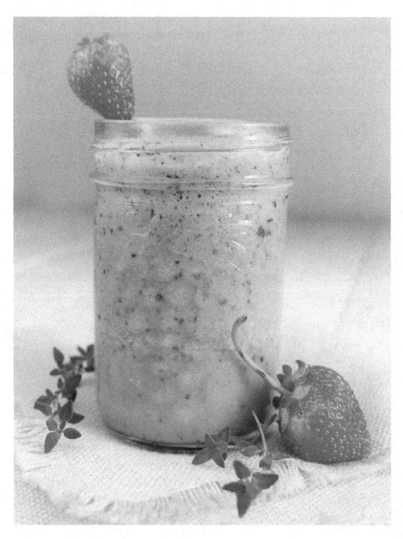

Total Prep & Cooking Time: Ten minutes

Yields: Two servings

Nutrition Facts: Calories: 301.9 | Protein: 5.4g | Carbs: 70.7g | Fat: 4.3g | Fiber: 8.9g

Ingredients

For the orange layer:

- One persimmon (quartered)
- One ripe mango (chopped)
- One lime (juiced)
- One tbsp. of nut butter (of your choice)
- Half tsp. of turmeric powder
- One pinch of cayenne pepper
- One cup of coconut milk

For the pink layer:

- One small beet (cubed)
- One cup of berries (frozen)
- One pink grapefruit (quartered)
- One-fourth cup of pomegranate juice
- Half cup of water
- Six leaves of mint
- One tsp. of honey

Method:

1. Add the ingredients for the orange layer in a blender. Blend for making a smooth liquid.

2. Pour the orange liquid evenly in serving glasses.

3. Add the pink layer ingredients in a blender. Blend for making a smooth liquid.

4. Pour the pink liquid slowly over the orange layer.

5. Pour in such a way so that both layers can be differentiated.

6. Serve immediately.

Total Prep & Cooking Time: Forty minutes

Yields: Two servings

Nutrition Facts: Calories: 140 | Protein: 2.6g | Carbs: 30.2g | Fat: 2.2g | Fiber: 5.6g

Ingredients

For carrot juice:

- Two cups of water
- Two and a half cups of carrots

For smoothie:

- One ripe banana (sliced)
- One cup of pineapple (frozen, cubed)
- Half tbsp. of ginger
- One-fourth tsp. of turmeric (ground)
- Half cup of carrot juice
- One tbsp. of lemon juice
- One-third cup of almond milk

Method:

1. Add water and carrots in a high power blender. Blend on high settings for making smooth juice.

2. Take a dish towel and strain the juice over a bowl. Squeeze the towel for taking out most of the juice.

3. Add the ingredients for the smoothie in a blender and blend until frothy and creamy.

4. Add carrot juice and blend again.

5. Pour the smoothie in glasses and serve.

Romaine Mango Smoothie

Total Prep & Cooking Time: Five minutes

Yields: Two servings

Nutrition Facts: Calories: 117.3 | Protein: 2.6g | Carbs: 30.2g | Fat: 0.9g | Fiber: 4.2g

Ingredients

- Sixteen ounces of coconut water
- Two mangoes (pitted)
- One head of romaine (chopped)
- One banana
- One orange (peeled)
- Two cups of ice

Method:

1. Add mango, romaine, orange, and banana in a high power blender. Blend the ingredients until frothy and smooth.

2. Add coconut water and ice cubes. Blend for one minute.

3. Pour the prepared smoothie in glasses and serve.

Fig Zucchini Smoothie

Total Prep & Cooking Time: Ten minutes

Yields: Two servings

Nutrition Facts: Calories: 243.3 | Protein: 14.4g | Carbs: 74.3g | Fat: 27.6g | Fiber: 9.3g

Ingredients

- Half cup of cashew nuts
- One tsp. of cinnamon (ground)
- Two figs (halved)
- One banana
- Half tsp. of ginger (minced)
- One-third tsp. of honey
- One-fourth cup of ice cubes
- One pinch of salt
- Two tsps. of vanilla extract
- Three-fourth cup of water
- One cup of zucchini (chopped)

Method:

1. Add all the listed ingredients in a high power blender. Blend for two minutes until creamy and smooth.

2. Pour the smoothie in serving glasses and serve.

Carrot Peach Smoothie

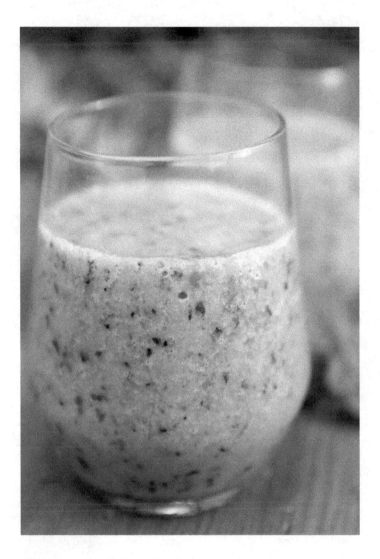

Total Prep & Cooking Time: Ten minutes

Yields: Two servings

Nutrition Facts: Calories: 191.2 | Protein: 11.2g | Carbs: 34.6g | Fat: 2.7g | Fiber: 5.4g

Ingredients

- Two cups of peach
- One cup of baby carrots
- One banana (frozen)
- Two tbsps. of Greek yogurt
- One and a half cup of coconut water
- One tbsp. of honey

Method:

1. Add peach, baby carrots, and banana in a high power blender. Blend on high settings for one minute.

2. Add Greek yogurt, honey, and coconut water. Give the mixture a whizz.

3. Pour the smoothie in glasses and serve.

Sweet Potato and Mango Smoothie
Total Prep & Cooking Time: Ten minutes

Yields: Two servings

Nutrition Facts: Calories: 133.3 | Protein: 3.6g | Carbs: 28.6g | Fat: 1.3g | Fiber: 6.2g

Ingredients

- One small sweet potato (cooked, smashed)
- Half cup of mango chunks (frozen)
- Two cups of coconut milk
- One tbsp. of chia seeds
- Two tsps. of maple syrup
- A handful of ice cubes

Method:

1. Add mango chunks and sweet potato in a high power blender. Blend until frothy and smooth.

2. Add chia seeds, coconut milk, ice cubes, and maple syrup. Blend again for one minute.

3. Divide the smoothie in glasses and serve.

Carrot Cake Smoothie

Total Prep & Cooking Time: Ten minutes

Yields: Two servings

Nutrition Facts: Calories: 289.3 | Protein: 3.6g | Carbs: 47.8g | Fat: 1.3g | Fiber: 0.6g

Ingredients

- One cup of carrots (chopped)
- One banana
- Half cup of almond milk
- One cup of Greek yogurt
- One tbsp. of maple syrup
- One tsp. of cinnamon (ground)
- One-fourth tsp. of nutmeg
- Half tsp. of ginger (ground)
- A handful of ice cubes

Method

1. Add banana, carrots, and almond milk in a blender. Blend until frothy and smooth.

2. Add yogurt, cinnamon, maple syrup, ginger, nutmeg, and ice cubes. Blend again for two minutes.

3. Divide the smoothie in serving glasses and serve.

Notes:

- You can add more ice cubes and turn the smoothie into slushy.

- You can store the leftover smoothie in the freezer for two days.

Chapter 4: Green Smoothies

Green smoothies can help in the process of detoxification as well as weight loss. Here are some easy-to-make green smoothie recipes for you.

Kale Avocado Smoothie

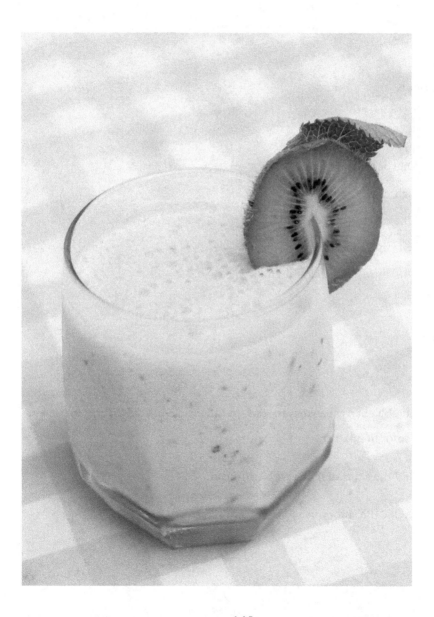

Total Prep & Cooking Time: Ten minutes

Yields: Two servings

Nutrition Facts: Calories: 401 | Protein: 11.2g | Carbs: 64.6g | Fat: 17.3g | Fiber: 10.2g

Ingredients

- One banana (cut in chunks)
- Half cup of blueberry yogurt
- One cup of kale (chopped)
- Half ripe avocado
- One-third cup of almond milk

Method:

1. Add blueberry, banana, avocado, and kale in a blender. Blend for making a smooth mixture.

2. Add the almond milk and blend again.

3. Divide the smoothie in glasses and serve.

Celery Pineapple Smoothie

Total Prep & Cooking Time: Ten minutes

Yields: Two servings

Nutrition Facts: Calories: 112 | Protein: 2.3g | Carbs: 3.6g | Fat: 1.2g | Fiber: 3.9g

Ingredients

- Three celery stalks (chopped)
- One cup of cubed pineapple
- One banana
- One pear
- Half cup of almond milk
- One tsp. of honey

Method:

1. Add celery stalks, pear, banana, and cubes of pineapple in a food processor. Blend until frothy and smooth.

2. Add honey and almond milk. Blend for two minutes.

3. Pour the smoothie in serving glasses and enjoy!

Cucumber Mango and Lime Smoothie

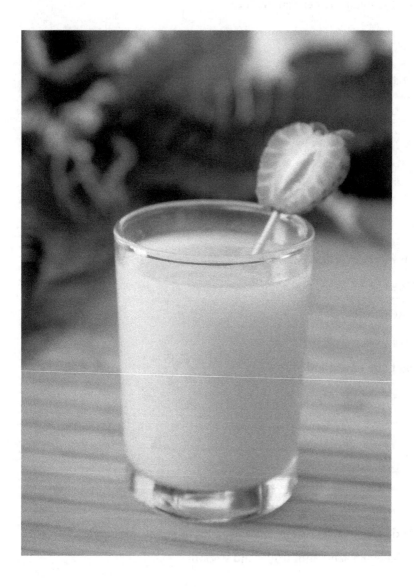

Total Prep & Cooking Time: Ten minutes

Yields: Two servings

Nutrition Facts: Calories: 165 | Protein: 2.2g | Carbs: 32.5g | Fat: 4.2g | Fiber: 3.7g

Ingredients

- One cup of ripe mango (frozen, cubed)
- Six cubes of ice
- Half cup of baby spinach leaves
- Two leaves of mint
- Two tsps. of lime juice
- Half cucumber (chopped)
- Three-fourth cup of coconut milk
- One-eighth tsp. of cayenne pepper

Method:

1. Add mango cubes, spinach leaves, and cucumber in a high power blender. Blend until frothy and smooth.

2. Add mint leaves, lime juice, coconut milk, cayenne pepper, and ice cubes. Process the ingredients until smooth.

3. Pour the smoothie in glasses and serve.

Kale, Melon, and Broccoli Smoothie

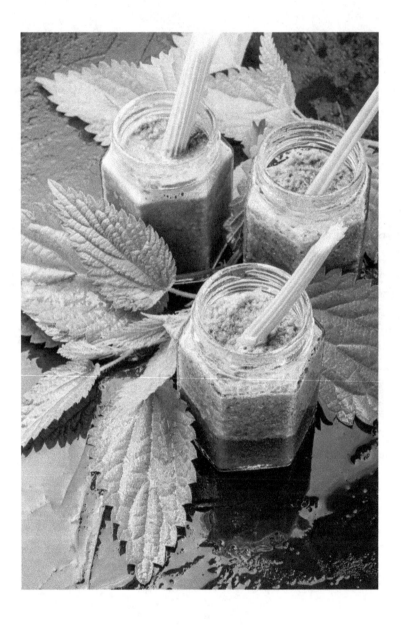

Total Prep & Cooking Time: Ten minutes

Yields: One serving

Nutrition Facts: Calories: 96.3 | Protein: 2.3g | Carbs: 24.3g | Fat: 1.2g | Fiber: 2.6g

Ingredients

- Eight ounces of honeydew melon
- One handful of kale
- Two ounces of broccoli florets
- One cup of coconut water
- Two sprigs of mint
- Two dates
- Half cup of lime juice
- Eight cubes of ice

Method:

1. Add kale, melon, and broccoli in a food processor. Whizz the ingredients for blending.

2. Add mint leaves and coconut water. Blend again.

3. Add lime juice, dates, and ice cubes. Blend the ingredients until smooth and creamy.

4. Pour the smoothie in a smoothie glass. Enjoy!

Kiwi Spinach Smoothie

Total Prep & Cooking Time: Ten minutes

Yields: Two servings

Nutrition Facts: Calories: 102 | Protein: 3.6g | Carbs: 21.3g | Fat: 2.2g | Fiber: 3.1g

Ingredients

- One kiwi (cut in chunks)
- One banana (cut in chunks)
- One cup of spinach leaves
- Three-fourth cup of almond milk
- One tbsp. of chia seeds
- Four cubes of ice

Method:

1. Add banana, kiwi, and spinach leaves in a blender. Blend the ingredients until smooth.

2. Add chia seeds, ice cubes, and almond milk. Blend again for one minute.

3. Pour the smoothie in serving glasses and serve.

Avocado Smoothie

Total Prep & Cooking Time: Ten minutes

Yields: Two servings

Nutrition Facts: Calories: 345 | Protein: 9.1g | Carbs: 47.8g | Fat: 16.9g | Fiber: 6.7g

Ingredients

- One ripe avocado (halved, pitted)
- One cup of milk
- Half cup of vanilla yogurt
- Eight cubes of ice
- Three tbsps. of honey

Method:

1. Add avocado, vanilla yogurt, and milk in a blender. Blend the ingredients until frothy and smooth.

2. Add honey and ice cubes. Blend the ingredients for making a smooth mixture.

3. Serve immediately.

PART V

Chapter 1: How to Choose the Right Number of Repetitions

"How do I choose the number of repetitions and series?"

This is one of the main doubts that assail the neophytes of the gym. I still remember the day I asked my gym instructor about it many years ago. In fact, the first questions that a beginner poses to the instructor in front of a weight machine are typically these: "How many consecutive lifts (or movements) do I have to do with this machines? And for how many times?"

The most precise ones even dare to ask how much time they have to recover from one set to the next one, and so you think you have clarified everything you need to know about a training session at a given weight machine.

The load (i.e., the kg lifted or moved) is generally fixed according to the presumed abilities of the aspiring visitor of the weight room, often without any relation to the first two parameters of repetitions and sets.

There is not a unique answer to these questions since it all depends on the goal. For example, when I first started my training journey, I wanted to get bigger, not stronger. During that period I did a lot of hypertrophy-oriented workouts which worked quite well. When I switched to a more strength-oriented approach, I had to completely rearrange my schedule all over again.

Since the weight training that interests us is not aimed at the practice of bodybuilding—but is framed in the health of those who want to integrate aerobic activities with exercises for the general improvement of strength, elasticity, and flexibility—before defining the number of repetitions and sets, it is necessary to establish the objective to be achieved or what aspect do you want to train for between the following:

- **The resistant force**: the force that the muscle must apply to overcome the fatigue resulting from a prolonged effort.

- **The maximal force**: the maximum force that the muscle can develop with a lifting test (or a limited number of tests). It is also often referred to as a maximal load if referring to a specific exercise in the gym.

- **The fast force:** the maximum force that the muscle can develop to counteract a load in a limited period of time. Referring to time, therefore, more than force we should speak of power which is the ability to develop a force in the unity of time.

- **Muscle hypertrophy**: no reference is made to the type of force that the muscle has to generate, but to its effect on the athlete's body—that is, to maximize the increase in muscle volume. The muscular volume is connected to the developed force, because the greater the cross section of the muscle, the greater the muscle fibers available to make the effort. However, the equation *muscle hypertrophy = greater muscle strength* is not always true because, in addition to having available muscle fibers, the human body must also know how to recruit, and this is influenced by other factors such as the efficiency of the cardio-respiratory system, the ability coordination, etc. This should make those who seek to maximize muscle hypertrophy think only of achieving the highest possible performance.

In a healthy view of strength training, you can leave out the last point because the search for muscle hypertrophy, typical of bodybuilders, is far from our goals. Therefore, we can identify three types of training, each of which corresponds to a type of strength that you want to train and, consequently, to a pattern of repetitions-number of sets-interval between the different series.

Remember that to define a training plan, the following variables must be defined for each exercise (i.e., for each machine in the gym or exercise with weights):

- Repetition: it is the single gesture of weightlifting or athletic gesture that stresses the muscle or a district of the muscles. Generally, in the gym at each repetition, the muscle or muscles lift or move a weight (load).

- Sets: the consecutive number of repetitions. The set can be slow or fast, or the exercise is done slowly, calmly, or quickly, imposing to adhere to a higher rhythm.

- Recovery: the time between one series and the next.

So, you might find a typical 3-row workout of 12 sets of 25 kg with a three-minute recovery. This is a very standard way to get started and the first style of training that I followed when started out.

Chapter 2: How to Breathe During Exercises

One thing that is often overlooked by many gym enthusiasts is how to perform proper breathing during weight exercises. It is a problem that, sooner or later, most of those who attend gyms propose to their instructor.

Breathing, as we know, is an activity that we do involuntarily, but it is also possible to control it trying to adapt the movement of the muscles (or part of the muscles) involved, such as the diaphragm, the ribcage, the shoulders, abdominals to the rhythm that we want to follow.

Consciously, one can control the inhalation phase and the exhalation phase in their overall duration or even suspend breathing by entering apnoea.

A lot of sports and disciplines (yoga, pilates, etc.), give a lot of importance to breathing, while other oriental disciplines even give it a spiritual value.

Even in the exercises that are performed in the gym, including those with weights, breathing has a considerable importance. Unfortunately, there are not many who have clear ideas about it.

Instructors usually advise to:

1 **inhale** in the discharge phase of the action, usually when the weight is being returned to its initial position;
2 **exhale** in the loading phase of the exercise or when there is more effort required.

This usually works well, even if the beginner will at first see this as another constraint which will only confuse him. In reality, it requires a good amount of concentration to force yourself to control breathing in this way and therefore forces the athlete to give complete attention to what he is doing. A lot of times, people look around in the gym while doing an exercise, or—worse—talking to someone. This is something that I have never understood: to me, strength training is a way to become the best version of myself, both physically and mentally, and I do not have time to waste. Focusing on breathing is a good way to think exclusively about the exercise you are performing.

The following is a good general rule to follow:

The most important thing to do is not to hold your breath during the loading phase.

Holding your breath in the loading phase is a big mistake, as it is instinctive to hold your breath during the maximum effort required. Instead, the opposite must be done because this practice can also lead to serious consequences, especially if the effort involves muscles of the upper body.

Holding the breath deliberately blocks the glottis, which then leads to a compression of the veins due to an increase in pressure inside the ribcage. As a result of this compression, the veins can also partially occlude (as if they were strangled by one hand) and this considerably slows the return of venous blood to the heart. As a consequence, the arterial pressure rises, reaching even impressive values such as 300 mmHg (usually 120 mmHg at rest). Moreover, as a consequence of the reduced blood supply to the heart, the outgoing blood also slows down and reduces, which decreases the blood and oxygen supply to the peripheral organs. Less blood and oxygen to the brain could result in dizziness, blurred vision, etc. until you eventually faint. These are side effects well-known by opera singers who practice hyperventilation exercises that, in some parts, are performed in apnoea.

Chapter 3: Machines or Free Weights?

The question is interesting, and the purpose of this chapter is to precisely evaluate the advantages and disadvantages of two possible training solutions for muscle strengthening: the use of gym machines or exercise with the aid of free weights.

From a health point of view, it is clear that the question of the title seems reasonable because, unlike in a bodybuilder, muscle strengthening is seen only as a preparatory to a sport or as a general improvement of the body, and therefore it is not said that the use of gym machines is actually the only possible solution for those who want to make a good upgrade without wanting to reach professional levels of a bodybuilding lover. Before analyzing the two solutions in detail, briefly remember that a muscle can perform an effort in two ways of contraction: eccentric or concentric.

In the first case, the muscle develops the force necessary for the exercise when it is stretching, in the second case when it is being shortened.

Weights and machines are not always equivalent in stimulating a muscle in an eccentric and concentric way. For the purpose of training, eccentric work is the most difficult—to the point that it can also induce pain and muscle damage. It is therefore important that, by deciding which exercises to perform (with the machines or with the weights), it is clear (otherwise you can ask the instructor like I did at the beginning of my journey in the gym) which exercises stimulate the muscles more eccentrically, to introduce them gradually into the plan of training avoiding injuries.

Weight Machines
In the gym, there are usually many weight machines. Generally, except for the

multi-function stations, each of them trains a specific muscular district or even a single type of muscle. The effort put in place by the muscles during the execution of the exercise must counteract two physical forces: the weight force and the force due to the friction of the weight that it moves (often along ropes or pulleys).

As a general rule of the mechanics involved in the use of weights, during the eccentric contraction, the friction force is subtracted from that of the weight, while during the concentric contraction this force is added.

Free Weights

They are called free-weight exercises because usually the weights are not tied to ropes or pulleys of the machines, but simply gripped or tied to the body (for example with anklets) and carried out only with the aid of weights such as dumbbells and barbells, which are often seen on sale in supermarkets. Surely, compared to a workout with machines, the one with free weights is easier to put in place. Often, it is not even necessary to attend a gym; a small home space equipped with a mat, a bench (if required by the exercises), a mirror (optional, to control the movements) and, of course, the weights is sufficient enough.

Now let's analyze the advantages and disadvantages of the two solutions, taking into consideration some objective parameters that can assume different importance depending on the individual's objectives, the physical state of departure (sedentary, beginner or advanced athlete), and the expectations placed in a training of this type.

1. Economic aspect: free weight training is certainly cheaper, because, as mentioned, in most cases it is not necessary to get a gym subscription. It can be a good compromise solution to go to the gym for the time necessary to practice the exercises under the guidance of an experienced

instructor, and then, once you are sure to perform the correct movements, buy weights and equip yourself with a training-space inside your home. This is what I did, and I would never go back.

2. Versatility: free weights are suitable for multiple exercises and different muscle groups. Think about how many exercises you can do with simple weights to train biceps, triceps, pectorals, etc. In the case of training with weight machines, each machine usually allows a few exercises (if not only one) and this is the practical limit of such a training: you need to choose a gym where there is a sufficient number of machines for the exercises you want to do and where waiting times are not too long. Otherwise, the queues to the machines make the overall workout boring and ineffective.

3. Eccentric and concentric training: weight machines usually lesser stress the eccentric work of the muscle (because of the opposing frictional force) unlike the movement of the body which, in returning to the starting position of the exercise, often performs eccentric work of considerable intensity. Moreover, in the exercises with weights, many antagonistic muscles are trained many times, and in general, they also train the balance and proprioceptive, improving body coordination.

4. Safety and complexity: from the previous point, we can see that weight machines train specific muscle areas, and it is easier to isolate the muscle or muscle district involved. It is also easier to perform the exercise correctly because the movements are constrained by the machines and are easier to learn. With free weights, it is easier to make mistakes, and generally more antagonistic muscles and the spine are stimulated. In addition, with the weights, it is easier to maintain a constant execution speed. For all these reasons, it is generally said that the exercises with the

machines are at a lower risk of injury than those with free weights.

Chapter 4: Putting it all together. How to program a training cycle?

Now we come to the crucial point: how do I craft a strength training program? The question is very complex. Each strategy will be based on the condition of the subject, so, logically, when we see a disproportionate lack of strength for a muscle group, it will be logical to intervene in this sense. Let's go step by step. The literature on the subject highlights how, for the purposes of muscular hypertrophy and gains in strength, setting a periodized program is the best solution. Before diving deeper into the topic, it is important to note something. You cannot generalize, there is no way to use a unique approach or way of training a particular component. There are countless cases, solutions. So what can be done is to report different models based on different contexts to give not a guide but a concept—something infinitely more precious (and expendable).

Strategy 1. "Basic" Approach. A first approach that we can use is to set up a multifrequency workout by adopting a daily wavy periodization. So we will have two weekly sessions for each muscle district. In the first session we can train the muscle according to a traditional bodybuilding scheme, then longer TUT, intensity techniques, a range of 8-12 repetitions, eccentric, forced, etc. In the second session, we can train ourselves by adopting a progression of strength. So for example, we will train the chest on a flat bench using possibly another complementary exercise (like crosses, chest fly, etc.). A similar approach is at the base of the PHAT (Power Hypertrophy Adaptive Training) method proposed by Norton. Unlike this, however, I find it more sensible to use—in training dedicated to strength—real progressions on exercises without being limited to a 5 × 5 standard type of training.

Strategy 2. Deficient Muscles Approach. Similar to the previous one, the only

164

difference is that a workout in this sense will be done on the deficient muscles while the more developed muscles will be trained in mono-frequency. The increase in weekly volume and stimulus variation will bring an advantage in terms of growth (strength and hypertrophy) that will allow you to "catch up" with respect to the rest of the muscles. This approach can be used on deficient muscles both from a hypertrophy point of view and from a force point of view (i.e., the weakest muscles). This last aspect is particularly important as it can be a valid strategy to intervene where a muscle is placed limiting within the synergy of a gesture. The discourse can also be done from the opposite point of view—that is, to hold the strongest or most developed muscle groups to a multifrequency and to mono-frequency to recover asymmetries (aesthetic or functional).

Strategy 3. The transient phase of reduced volume. Another way to insert a strength training within a bodybuilding program is to provide a period with a high load intensity and a reduced volume. In this case, we always speak of wavy periodization. However, the variations will not be done on a daily basis, but weekly. So, for instance, we will put 2-3 up to 6 weeks of strength training with a reduced volume—less dense workouts but with the intensity of high-load and then return, progressively or not, to traditional bodybuilding sessions, or even to a wavy periodization protocol on a daily basis as described above. Basically, it is a matter of setting a transitional phase aimed at two purposes: Varying the stimulus (Ri) and finding the feeling with the motor scheme.

Strategy 4. Periodization within the session. This is also an interesting approach. It is a matter of inserting, within the session, an exercise on which to set up a forced schedule. In this sense, we could then insert the flat bench into a chest session as a first or second exercise. We will choose a program to improve on strength (since we are already able to exercise the right mastery over the exercise) and set the rest of the session as a traditional bodybuilding session. Obviously, the total volume will decrease as part of the session is occupied by dense work—not very voluminous but very intense. I find that such a setting fits well with the daily wavy periodization (strategy 1). Basically, by training a multi-frequency muscle, we will set the strength session using an exercise with its progression and the rest of the session in the traditional bodybuilding style. The diversification of work with respect to the second weekly session will be in the TUT (for example) which, in the latter, will be exasperated (e.g., +50'), while in the session of "strength" it will not be too high (e.g., 30').

Split and choice of exercises

A further aspect on which we must dwell is that relative to the decision, within the session, the target muscle groups and the exercises to be used. One of the characteristics of strength programs is that, in most cases, the various muscle groups are subdivided to work only a few each session. This is logical because the work that is required is always of the same type (anaerobic). Okay, as we have seen, it can work on different adaptive components, but in any case, it is always part of the big family of "boosting" work, the same that, in other sports, is alternated with "technical" work. The question that arises is the following: Should we first set the split and then, based on this, choose the type of exercises in which to work the strength or vice versa? Being a powerlifter myself, I would answer "the second," but from a Bodybuilder perspective I would answer "the first." Since this chapter is about strength training, I would say start from this context and, in particular, from the cases mentioned above. Where we want to set a wavy periodization, for all groups or only for some (strategies 1-2-4), then yes, we will have to start from the split. Based on this we will choose the best exercise on which to progress for the strength. So for example, in a push-day, we will choose the Bench Press for the chest, for a pull-day a Bent Over Row, and for a leg-day a Squat.

Let's do an example: Subject 1, Powerlifter, good management of high loads on the various motor schemes. Deficient groups: Arms, Back. Strong groups: Chest, Quadriceps

Split

Day 1 Push Day

Day 2 Pull Day

Day 3 Leg Day

Day 4 Rest

Day 5 Arms

Day 6 Back

Day 7 Glutes

Logically, we will then insert a progression on the Bent-Over Row on day 2 and work the Back with a traditional strength session on day 6. To evaluate a progression on the ground clearance that would be close to a leg workout (even putting it on day 6), we will have the hamstrings on day 7. But training strength, as we have seen, is not just a matter of periodizing and varying the stimulus, but also a question of functionality to the motor schemes to be performed during the sessions.

So let's take another example. Subject 2: Powerlifter, poor activation of the chest on the bench press, poor feeling on the deadlift. Excellent management of the Squat. Deficient groups: Chest-Back-Arms. The goal, in this case, will be to improve the feeling with easier exercises so we will set the split based on the same.

Split

Day 1 Chest and Shoulders

Day 2 Deadlift day

Day 3 Rest

Day 4 Quadriceps and Arms

Day 5 Rest

Day 6 Chest and Back

Day 7 Arms

Finally, in case we go set up a Strength program as a transitory phase (strategy 3), it will be logical to start from the exercises and, based on these, reason on the split.